The Daily T...

DEPRESSION
What You Really Need to Know

The Daily Telegraph

DEPRESSION
What You Really Need to Know

DR VIRGINIA EDWARDS

ROBINSON
London

Constable & Robinson Ltd
3 The Lanchesters
162 Fulham Palace Road
London W6 9ER
www.constablerobinson.com

First published in Canada by Key Porter Books Limited, 2002

First published in the UK by Robinson,
an imprint of Constable & Robinson Ltd, 2003

Consultant to the UK edition: Dr Meredith Duke

Publisher's Note: This book is not intended to be a substitute for medical
advice or treatment. Any person with a condition requiring medical
attention should consult a qualified medical practitioner
or suitable therapist.

ISBN 1-84119-806-4

Printed and bound in Great Britain by Bookmarque Ltd

10 9 8 7 6 5 4 3 2 1

Contents

Foreword

There are few more dramatic, or gratifying, opportunities for family doctors to change the lives of their patients for the better than the modern treatment of depression with its capacity to restore, in just a few weeks, the miserable and dejected back to their normal selves. Indeed doctors have come to believe so strongly in the value of their treatment they now write an astonishing 13 million more prescriptions for antidepressant drugs every year than just a decade ago, which means there are now approximately 3 million regular users in Britain every day. And for those who might feel this is overdoing it, a survey from Australia shows there to be a direct causal link between this general trend of the rising number of prescriptions and the steep decline in those seeking to take their own lives.

And yet, as Dr Virginia Edwards points out in her lucid guide to this devastating, but eminently treatable condition, there are, it would seem, still many for whom its recognition is unnecessarily delayed or whose therapy is insufficiently rigorous or prolonged. Depression comes in many different guises: it can be episodic or continuous, it may be precipitated by grief or loss, or be part of a person's psychological makeup; it may be mild or severe – but the major insight of recent years has been how these are all points on a continuum of the same condition that ranges all the way from an exaggerated response to a stressful situation to incapacitating distress and disability.

It is very difficult for others to grasp the ordeal of the afflicted for which the poet Syliva Plath invoked the metaphor of a Bell Jar in her book of that name: the glass dome placed over fragile items to protect them catches the frightening combination of being both disconnected from the world and yet suffocated by it. Friends and relatives can, however, offer the only effective antidote – the 'hope' that such deeply ingrained pessimism is indeed reversible no matter how unlikely that might seem.

The two singular virtues of Dr Edwards' book is first the manner in which she catches in a series of case histories the variety of depression along its continuum, and then provides a clear perspective on the range of treatment options whether the talking cures of psychotherapy or drug medication.

The talking therapies have been revolutionized by the displacement of the time consuming and usually ineffective psychoanalytic approach as formulated by Sigmund Freud by the much more straightforward concepts of cognitive therapy. This, as its name implies, is concerned with what, or more precisely how, people think about themselves and the world around them. Thoughts exert a profound influence on feelings and so distorted patterns of thinking (such as the belief that life is pointless) can profoundly effect the emotion. In cognitive therapy these distorted patterns of thinking are identified and, in theory, once corrected, the feelings they cause of depression and anxiety should be ameliorated.

The rise of cognitive therapy in recent years has been complemented by the introduction of an ever-wider range of drugs that act on the neurotransmitters in the brain. The precise mechanism as to why these drugs – of which the best known is probably Prozac – influence mental states remains elusive, and may always be so. But the only important thing, from a practical perspective, is that they work. They may not do so for everybody or they can have some adverse effects whose seriousness has only recently been realized. Nonetheless there are now seven different types, so it should be possible by a process of trial and error to find the most appropriate.

I sincerely hope that those reading this book will find for themselves – or those they care for – the means to shift the clouds of despondency and so let the sun shine through again.

Introduction

Anna, fifty years old, says, 'I feel tense and guilty but I don't know why. I can't sleep or eat, so my friends have to come over to feed me. Even when I do get some sleep, I'm so exhausted when I wake up that I can't get out of bed. I'm terrified about what's happening to me.'

Adult depression is a common illness. One in five people will have a depressive illness during their lifetime. Twice as many women as men are affected. Unfortunately, over half the cases are not diagnosed, let alone treated. This is partly because, at the beginning, the problems don't seem different from the sadness or low moods that we all feel from time to time. When someone develops a high blood-sugar level, as in diabetes, or breaks a leg, there's a distinct onset or difference we can pinpoint that says the person has the illness. In depression, it's a question of the severity of the feelings, and the length of time the person feels bad. But even though the onset is not apparent, treatment is important. Work life, social life, and intimate relationships all suffer. The affected person loses interest in other people, feels exhausted and hopeless, and wants to give up. In fact, when the illness is untreated and severe, the risk of successful suicide can be as high as 15 per cent.

Since 1960, research into the causes and treatment of depression has greatly increased. We now know that in the majority of cases depression can be treated effectively. However, despite the breakthroughs in knowledge and treatment, stigma and embarrassment still surround the illness. It is difficult to admit you can't manage your life. In addition, friends, employers, and even family members are frightened by the changes they see, leaving you more isolated at the very time you need support and reassurance. You may be reluctant to ask for the help you need.

Old prejudices die hard. In a recent survey looking at the public perception of the causes of depressive illness, 71 per cent of respondents felt it was due to emotional weakness, 45 per cent felt it was the victim's fault, and 35 per cent thought it was due to sinful behaviour.

In fact, depression is a serious medical illness, causing more disability than any other disorder except advanced coronary artery disease. Untreated depression affects every aspect of your life. Accidents, suicide attempts, substance abuse, family dysfunction, and poor work performance are all common. Yet depression responds to treatment in over 80 per cent of cases. The other 20 per cent will show a partial response, or require different treatment methods. The greatest barriers to taking advantage of treatment are denial and embarrassment.

Sarah had been a hard-working, conscientious employee in the accounts department of a large clothing manufacturer.

She seldom missed a day's work and always had the month-end figures ready and balanced. She began to feel tired and worn out just after celebrating her forty-fifth birthday. At first, she thought she was under too much stress.

Her husband, Michael, had lost his job and was earning only half his previous income, as a self-employed consultant. Sarah worried constantly because they were somewhat overextended on their credit cards. She would wake up suddenly at four in the morning with her heart pounding and her body perspiring. Her thoughts would spin as she tried to sort out her problems, and she wouldn't get back to sleep. She was tired and irritable at work, and started falling behind. Michael made dinner each evening because she was too exhausted. She would lie down in the bedroom, ignoring him and their two young sons. She even refused to go to the cinema at the weekend, as they had done in the past.

As her fears and lack of energy escalated, she became alarmed and told Michael that she thought she was going crazy. Though he was beginning to wonder himself, he told her not to be silly. He said she just had to stop worrying and try to enjoy herself. He thought a visit to her out-of-town sister might cheer her up. Sarah did visit her sister, but she came back from the trip feeling worse than ever. Exasperated, Michael told her to stop feeling sorry for herself, and Sarah became more withdrawn and morose, overcome by how useless she felt.

Sarah's work deteriorated as she came home early to sleep. She no longer helped the boys with their homework. Her appetite diminished and she lost weight, though she was already slim. She hardly spoke to Michael or the boys but spent long periods alone.

Finally Michael became alarmed, thinking she might have

a serious illness. He made an appointment for her to see their family doctor, and insisted she go with him. Fortunately, their family doctor had known them for years, and realized how morose and irritable Sarah had become. The doctor did a physical examination and a number of blood tests, as well as an electrocardiogram, to rule out physical illness.

Once their doctor had the results, she sat down with both Sarah and Michael and told them what she thought was happening: Sarah was fine physically but was suffering from a major depression. She said Sarah needed to take some time off work, to ease up on her expectations of herself, and to begin talking about her feelings to Michael and her doctor. She also said that they might consider an antidepressant medication that had helped other people with similar illnesses.

Both Sarah and Michael felt relieved once they had an explanation for what was happening. They decided to take their doctor's advice. They also found out all they could about the illness, by reading and by searching the Internet.

Sarah started taking the antidepressants and, although the side effects were somewhat uncomfortable, she persevered. Within three or four weeks she started to feel better and had more energy. She also began sleeping better. In the meantime, because she was unable to complete work assignments, and was worried that she might lose her job, her doctor wrote a letter to her employer.

Fortunately, Sarah's illness was recognized early and treated well. But she was fortunate her family doctor recognized her condition. About 50 per cent of cases are misdiagnosed at this stage. Even when the illness is recognized, it is only treated adequately in about half the cases. Because of popular prejudice, and the depressed person's negative attitude, many people are less able to find the help they need.

The cost in personal distress, work disability, and social isolation can be compared to that of other serious, chronic, and recurrent health conditions, such as diabetes, heart disease, and high blood pressure. In any one year, 9.5 per cent of the population will experience depression serious enough to destroy their enjoyment of living. The World Health Organization predicts that by 2020 depression will be the leading cause of disease and disability globally. At some time in their lives, 20 per cent of the population will suffer depression. Yet 66 per cent of countries devote one per cent or less of their health-care budget to treatment of depression.

The chief purpose of this book is to provide information so you or your loved ones can get the best help possible. The following chapters will help you become an informed consumer. If you're very depressed it is sometimes difficult to absorb new information, or even to find the energy to read. Don't worry. This ability is lost only temporarily. As your mood improves, you'll be able to learn more about your illness.

It is also important that family and friends learn about the nature of the illness, so they can help. The symptoms can be mystifying to them, as they aren't sure what's happening.

In most cases, the illness does improve. As well, you'll be better able to manage if you're well informed. Support is available and it works. The more you know about the illness, the less prejudice and fear will interfere with you or your loved ones receiving effective help.

1
Depression: Normal and Abnormal

Raj is forty years old, and has recurrent major depressive episodes. 'Why do I have to suffer so much?' he asks. 'All the things I can't do, the plans I can't make, because I don't know what shape I'll be in from one week to the next. For the last two days I haven't cared about anything, I haven't even taken a shower. I've just been trying to manage the pain of my own emotions. Tonight at supper I started to feel sane, and then the despair hit me again, like a ton of bricks. I'm afraid one of these days my boss will fire me. How do I get healthy, and stay that way?'

We all experience feelings and emotions. These are signals that tell us if we are safe or in danger. They also communicate to others that we are upset or pleased. We can cope with changes in the world by tuning into our feelings, the signalling system that sends emotional messages that are universally recognizable, and interprets other people's emotions accurately. Feelings are the subjective awareness of emotions.

In fact, feelings are present throughout mammalian species. Dogs and gorillas can signal happiness by jumping playfully and showing their teeth, much as humans do when they smile. The physical signs of the emotion, such as a smile, a grimace, a red face, clenched fists, or downcast eyes, indicate the state we're in to those around us. Although we are not always conscious of what we communicate, the signals we send, such as a raised voice, a cry, or a hunched posture, tell other people what responses we need from them. Sometimes we don't have time to think what to do in response. A stranger hears the distressed cry of someone drowning and, without thinking, jumps in to save the person. When the stranger is given a medal for heroism, he or she says there was no conscious act of bravery.

The more varied our awareness and expression of our feelings, the healthier we are emotionally. Healthy families accept and encourage the expression and awareness of a full range of feelings in their children. They accept the children's anger, sadness, and joyfulness. They neither deny nor censor these feelings, although this doesn't mean the child is allowed to act in a hurtful way. Healthy families also accept other people's faults, and enjoy being with others. They are sociable and outgoing.

That's the ideal. Most of us manage to approach it rather than achieve it. I can remember self-righteously criticizing someone for being bitter, only to realize the next day that I had been the negative one. Good therapy helps us relax our rigidity so we can experience the full range and richness of feelings. We need to feel angry, sad, happy, joyful, and a whole range of more subtle emotions to feel truly alive.

Moods versus Depression

A mood is a state of emotion sustained for a period of time. When we're in a 'good mood' we feel buoyant, self-confident, and happy. We're interested in what's happening around us and want to explore new things. Usually something good has happened to us or we are having fun with people we like. We feel positive about ourselves and optimistic about the state of the world. Pity we can't feel this way all the time! But if we did, we'd miss out on signs of danger.

'Bad moods' start when we feel anxious, angry, frightened, or sad. Often these feelings are provoked by some external event – not getting the promotion we wanted, finding out we're overdrawn at the bank, or, worse yet, learning that our company is downsizing or our partner is fed up and thinking of leaving the relationship. If we didn't feel anxious, irritable, sad, or frightened under these circumstances, we wouldn't be able to look out for our needs. We have to be able to take steps to protect ourselves from hurt and humiliation so we can survive adversities and maintain our self-esteem.

The word 'depressed' can describe a feeling, as in 'I'm so depressed that John didn't call for a date for Saturday night.' It can also convey a more persistent state of low mood, as in 'I've felt so depressed since I found out I was passed over for the promotion I'd worked so hard for, and I can't shake it.' Usually, when we experience the feeling or mood as appropriate and understandable, we don't rush off to a doctor. We know we will cheer up when things change, or we look for other ways to handle our disappointments.

Feeling blue, sad, defeated, depleted, or helpless is all part of being human. We experience these feelings when things go wrong in our world. Paradoxically, if we don't accept these

---

Disorders and degrees

If you think about it, some other illnesses are like depression, in that they are defined by an excessive degree of what would otherwise be normal. For example, high blood pressure is a condition of the blood pressure being persistently above normal, and the higher it is, the more it needs treatment. Obesity refers to a weight level significantly above average, and greater obesity is more serious. It's the same for depression. The level of severity determines when treatment is necessary.

---

feelings – if we're rigid and controlled – we experience even more emotional distress. Our energy gets used up in suppressing the feelings and denying the hurt. We give up but we don't know why. At this point, the illness of depression can result.

How Depressed Is Depressed?

Depression can be distinguished from sadness in a number of ways. The intensity of the sadness is more severe and painful. A sufferer may describe the pain as 'worse than any physical pain'. The pain is so unbearable that often you feel you would rather be dead. The sadness pervades all aspects of your life and can't be shaken off. The feeling takes on a life of its own; it seems detached from whatever the original painful event was, so that you can't be reasoned out of the horrible feelings. You feel guilty and worthless and reproach yourself for your failings. You are unable to express your feelings or experience any pleasure. You have difficulty concentrating, feel unpleasant body sensations, are agitated or slowed down, and appear downcast and unsmiling.

The above paragraph describes clinical depression. Several scales have been developed so that the doctor can assign a number value measuring the severity of the depression; these scales also give you a way to see if the depression is improving with treatment.

The Patient Health Questionnaire

Simple screening tests such as the Patient Health Questionnaire pick up many cases. If at least five of the following nine descriptions apply to you, and if these symptoms are increasing in frequency and severity over a two-week period, you are likely have a depressive illness that should be treated. If your depression needs to be treated, you are unable to function in many areas of your life. You are impaired at home, at work, and with friends. If you have actively thought about suicide, you would be wise to get help as soon as possible.

- little interest or pleasure in doing things
- feeling down, depressed, or hopeless
- trouble falling or staying asleep, or sleeping too much
- feeling tired or having little energy
- poor appetite or overeating
- feeling bad about yourself, or feeling that you are a failure or have let yourself or your family down
- trouble concentrating while reading the newspaper or watching television
- moving or speaking so slowly that other people would notice, or the opposite – being so fidgety or restless that you can't stop moving
- thinking that you would be better off dead, or thinking of hurting yourself in some way

If you have only two or three of these symptoms, you should

view them as a warning. Talking over your feelings and concerns with someone who cares about you may help. You could also lighten up on the demands you make on yourself, spending less time working and more time enjoying yourself, although this isn't always possible. Looking after yourself with comfortable sleep, exercise, and nutritious food, and spending time with friends and family, can also help. If the feelings don't let up, you should see a doctor or counsellor to talk over your problems.

If you have more than four of these feelings or have suicidal thoughts, it's important to seek help from your doctor or a counsellor. Lots of good help is available. You might start by seeing your family doctor. If the doctor feels you are depressed, he or she may decide to treat you personally with medication, or may refer you to a counsellor or psychiatrist, a medical specialist with several years of additional training in treating psychiatric illness.

Some health plans will pay for these services. Most general hospitals have a mental health clinic where people with depressive disorders can be treated. A psychologist or social worker, professionals trained in counselling people with depressive illnesses, may be assigned to treat you. You can be treated free by your local NHS (National Health Service) or, if you have private health insurance, by private psychiatric and psychotherapy services. Different insurance schemes offer different degrees of cover for in-patient care, day care and psychotherapy/counselling/support services. Psychologists and social workers work as therapists in private practice as well. In the UK these services may be covered by insurance plans and some company health plans will pay for a designated number of sessions. Some psychotherapy services offer sliding-scale fees for people with limited resources who are prepared to pay towards their own treatment. You local psychiatric services or family doctor can put you in touch with these services.

The Hamilton Psychiatric Rating Scale

A more thorough scale for determining the severity of depressive illness is called the Hamilton Psychiatric Rating Scale for Depression. Dr Max Hamilton first developed this test in 1960. Since then it has become a benchmark for measuring the level of depression. The Hamilton Scale has twenty-one categories with two to four ranges of severity. The categories are wide-ranging and include depressed mood, guilt feelings, sleep disturbances, weight loss, anxiety, agitation, body ailments, suicidal thoughts, and impaired thinking. Your doctor scores the form and gives a numerical rating for you initially, and then tracks your improvement with treatment. A score of 7 or less indicates no illness. A score between 13 and 17 usually indicates a treatable illness called dysthymia, explained in Chapter 2. A score between 18 and 25 indicates a major depressive disorder. A score between 26 and 30 shows a more severe form of depression called melancholia, and a score above 30 indicates very severe depression.

Another scale, the Beck Depression Inventory, is scored by the patient, and likewise indicates levels of severity.

Other Tests for Depression

You can see that depression is a continuum from an exaggerated response to stress to incapacitating distress and disability. Over the years, scientists have tried to find biological markers or consistent changes in the chemistry of the

Cortisone and depression

One early attempt to distinguish serious depression from normal stress response was the dexamethasone suppression test. The adrenal gland secretes a hormone called cortisone to help us deal with stress. Normally our blood cortisone level is highest around midnight and lowest around six a.m., and the adrenal gland's secretion of cortisone is suppressed if dexamethasone (a form of cortisone) is given. In severely depressed people the blood cortisone level stays high around the clock, and the adrenal gland keeps secreting cortisone even if dexamethasone is being administered. It was hoped that tracking the cortisone level with and without dexamethasone would identify people who needed help for their depression. Unfortunately, the results of the test are affected by factors such as diet and other illnesses, and the test is not reliable enough to be useful.

body that can be measured to distinguish between normal responses to stress, which the person will recover from spontaneously, and debilitating illnesses that will improve only with active treatment.

Often the first sign of a depressive episode is difficulty sleeping. The time between falling asleep and the onset of

Types of depression

Depressive disorders
- major depressive episode
- major depressive disorder
  - melancholia
  - psychotic depression
  - seasonal affective disorder
  - atypical depression
- dysthymia
- masked depression (somatization disorder)

Bipolar disorders
- bipolar I
- bipolar II
  - rapid cycling disorder
  - cyclothymic disorder

rapid eye movement (REM) sleep, otherwise known as dream sleep – when the eyeballs move rapidly – is shortened in someone who is depressed. A sleep lab taking an electroencephalogram (a test that shows brainwave patterns) during the night can determine if a person has a sleep pattern characteristic of depression. This method of deciding if someone has a treatable depression is too expensive to use routinely, but it's helpful and is used in centres where research in depression takes place.

In short, at the present time the diagnosis of depression is based on the amount of distress and disability the individual is suffering. Doctors and researchers hope that in the future they will find a measure that is simple and exact.

The next two chapters explain the different categories of depression more thoroughly. New names of syndromes have been added as the various categories were studied more thoroughly. Many terms overlap and can describe the same symptoms. Chapters 2 and 3 will clarify some of these terms.

2
Depressive Disorders

Janice, a forty-four-year-old full-time schoolteacher, visited her doctor's office complaining of fatigue, difficulty keeping up with the demands of her busy family of three children, lack of interest in sex with her husband, and irritable outbursts that were getting her into trouble at work and at home. 'Up until six months ago I was feeling all right, particularly during the summer holidays', she said. 'But things went downhill, and by February, I knew I needed help. I can't even sleep well. I keep waking up at four or five in the morning with a sick feeling in the pit of my stomach, as if I've done something terribly wrong.'

Janice's doctor asked if anything had happened six months ago. Janice couldn't recall anything very significant. She did remember being upset in June because of education cutbacks that meant she would have to work longer hours in a job that bored her. With her husband's business not doing as well as they had hoped, she couldn't afford to decrease her hours, and she admitted to being somewhat resentful about it.

Finally, though, something else came out. Janice said that her estranged father, who had left the family when she was eight because her mother could no longer tolerate his drinking, had come back into her life and was terminally ill. She remembered him being playful and fun when she was a little girl. He had always seemed to adore her, but she had seen very little of him after the breakup, and he had not helped with her expenses or schooling. Janice had had problems in her last year of university and had spent long periods in bed that winter, missing so many classes that she had almost failed. She had gone to the student health service but had been too embarrassed to talk about her problems.

Janice looked sad. Her eyes teared as she spoke, although she didn't cry, and she seemed restless and uncomfortable. She had no makeup on, her hair was unwashed, and there was a stain on her blouse. The doctor was concerned about her dishevelled appearance and her obvious unhappiness.

Janice's doctor began by getting as thorough a history as possible. The doctor let Janice tell her story in her own words, and went on to ask her when she had started feeling bad, what events such as life changes or illnesses had been going on at the time, if there were any medical illnesses or drug therapies that might coincide with the onset of her feeling low. How incapacitated had she become? Was she eating and sleeping? Was she able to get up and dressed in the morning? Was she still able to work? Did she still enjoy her regular activities in the evening? What had she tried to do so far to make herself feel better? And, most important, did she feel so bad that she'd lost hope and thought of killing herself?

The doctor also inquired about other bouts of psychiatric

illness, and any allied symptoms, such as panic attacks or obsessive-compulsive symptoms. 'Do you have a feeling as if something terrible is going to happen, and you break out in perspiration, and your heart starts beating fast? Do you find you can't leave the house without checking the cooker and the door over and over, or do you start to badger yourself about saying the wrong thing or not doing something you should have, and you can't let it go?' The doctor asked about physical ailments such as headache, chest pain, stomach pain, or excessive drinking. 'What sort of person were you before you became sick – were you outgoing and sociable or quiet and retiring?'

Then Janice's doctor looked for illness in the family. Had any relatives related by blood – such as mother, father, grandparents, aunts and uncles, brothers, sisters, children, nieces and nephews – been treated or hospitalized for depression or anxiety? Were there hints of suicides and alcoholism? In many families, these illnesses are kept secret out of embarrassment. The doctor also checked for less obvious symptoms. Were Janice's parents moody, outgoing, crotchety, withdrawn? Were they able to form relationships, hold down jobs, participate in the community? These are all signs of healthy functioning. The doctor asked about early losses, chronic illnesses, and neglect by her parents in childhood. Eventually, based on all this information and more, Janice was diagnosed as having a major depressive episode – a common and serious form of depression.

This may seem like a lot of information to ask someone who doesn't feel like talking, but people can be amazingly open when they first come for help. In many cases, the first session produces all the information the doctor needs for the rest of the therapy. The facts learned later are like commentary on the first session.

A good medical and physical examination is done to rule out any contributing medical illnesses. Ideally, the physical examination should be done by a doctor who won't be counselling the person. There are valid reasons for this. Many depressed people have had unpleasant and physically intrusive experiences with caregivers in the past, and the examination may feel invasive and uncomfortable. This option of different doctors is often not available, so the family doctor may do both the physical examination and the psychotherapy.

Major Depressive Episode

By definition, if you have a major depressive episode you have a depressed mood, marked by sadness, hopelessness, helplessness, and worthlessness, lasting for at least two weeks. You can't shake the gloomy feelings by talking to yourself. All areas of living are affected. Indecision, difficulty concentrating, fatigue, and loss of interest in life wear you down.

The mood is inappropriately low, and described by sufferers as 'psychic torment' or a 'dark night of the soul'. People who have been through a major depression say the pain is far worse than the worst physical pain. There can be severe agitation, so you pace up and down and can't rest. At other times, thoughts, speech, body movements, and facial expressions are slowed down. Feelings of guilt and worth-lessness out of proportion to any deeds torment you. You lose your appetite, so weight loss can be rapid. You wake alert and fearful at three or four in the morning and can't get back to sleep. Sexual interest is non-existent. Sufferers will tell you that the experience is distinct from and far worse than normal grief or loss. In fact, if untreated, 15 per cent of these people will eventually commit suicide.

The first bout of major depression usually lasts about six to nine months. In 50 to 60 per cent of people the illness recurs within a year. Once you have had one recurrence, the chances of further recurrences increase. If treatment does not return you to your original level of functioning, you may develop a chronic pattern of depressive symptoms. Complete remission – that is, an absence of symptoms – leads to fewer and less frequent recurrences. Early, thorough treatment can prevent a more chronic and debilitating disease.

A single bout of depression lasting six to nine months, with disabling symptoms, is called a depressive episode. If you have a recurrence or a repeat episode a few months to a few years later, you are said to be suffering from major depressive disorder.

Author William Styron wrote about his experiences with major depression eloquently in the book *Darkness Visible*. He described 'a howling tempest in the brain', 'dreadful, pouncing seizures of anxiety', 'a kind of numbness, an enervation, an odd fragility – as if my body had actually become frail, hypersensitive and somehow disjointed and clumsy'.

Sylvia Plath used the metaphor of a bell jar in her book about her experiences with the illness. The image of the bell jar – the glass dome placed over fragile items to protect them – catches the terrifying sense of feeling both disconnected and suffocated. The sufferer can't join with others and others can't reach her.

What Is Depressive Illness?

Historically, unipolar and bipolar depressions were seen as two distinct types of depressive disorders – affecting different groups of the population, requiring different treatments, and having different lifetime courses. Polar refers to which pole (extreme) of mood, either elated or depressed, the person is experiencing. The term 'unipolar depression' is no longer used.

People with depression experience only one extreme, the depressive pole in its different forms, during the course of the illness. They do not have elated or excited periods. In this chronic disorder the individual can be free of the illness for a time. Some people have only one episode and never experience a recurrence. Others are never totally disabled but neither do they feel totally well. People with bipolar illnesses experience both elated and depressed periods during the course of their illness. Your doctor cannot distinguish between depression and the depressive phase of bipolar disorder from the signs and symptoms in one episode. Bipolar illness has at least one episode of mania or hypomania, interspersed with recurrent depressive episodes. The course of the illness – the occurrence of one or both extremes – determines the type of illness. The types of depression described in this chapter are different presentations of depressive illness only. Bipolar illness is described in Chapter 3.

Types of Depressive Illness

Melancholia

Early in the twentieth century, depression was classified as either reactive or endogenous. Reactive depression was thought to be milder in nature, and caused by an outside event. Endogenous depression was considered more severe and was thought to begin spontaneously, without an external cause. Usually the person had weight loss and sleeping problems, slowed thinking, and agitation or retardation of movement. Another name for this type of depression is melancholia. This term captures the anguish of the sufferer better than the word 'depression'.

Both of these types – indeed, all the types of depression described in this chapter – are now thought to be different manifestations of the same disorder. The illness can change from mild to severe, sometimes has an external cause, and sometimes occurs spontaneously.

Psychotic Depression

In some cases, depression becomes so severe that the person develops delusions and hallucinations. ('Psychosis' means the person is out of touch with reality.) Delusions are frightening fixed ideas that are not open to argument. If you have a depressive delusion, you may think that you are already dead, or that you are responsible for all the evil in the world. Auditory hallucinations are usually experienced as disembodied voices telling you to kill yourself, or saying that you are worthless. Psychotic depression is an emergency situation, because the delusions and hallucinations are so compelling and real to you that you may feel forced to act on them.

Dysthymia

Martin is a hard-working executive in a small firm. He does most of the organizing and trouble-shooting in the office. He sets very high standards for himself and other employees, and can become irritable and sarcastic when these are not met. He knows he alienates people. Despite his bad temper, he's a valued employee who always runs the office efficiently.

Outside of work, Martin stays at home in the evenings to clean his flat or goes to the gym to work out. He would like to have more fun and go on dates. Unfortunately, he finds fault with his friends and the women he is introduced to. Eventually they start avoiding him.

Martin can't remember a time when he felt relaxed and happy. He is always anticipating trouble and worried about the future. He thinks other people must feel the same way but manage to hide it better.

Martin has a condition called dysthymic disorder, a chronic illness with less debilitating symptoms than major depression. About 6 per cent of the population is affected. This illness begins gradually, in people in their late teens or early twenties with a family history of depression. Life appears grey. The person experiences a depressed mood on most days of the week for at least two years, never being free of symptoms for more than two months. Symptoms include poor appetite or overeating, insomnia or oversleeping, low energy and fatigue, low self-esteem, poor concentration, and difficulty in making decisions, along with pessimistic feelings.

Dysthymia is a serious disorder with a chronic course. At a five-year follow-up of people with dysthymia, 76 per cent had gone on to develop a major depressive episode.

Dysthymia has only recently been recognized as treatable. The advent of newer and safer antidepressants means that people who have suffered from this disorder for years can actually begin to enjoy life, sometimes for the first time in many years. Previously, those with dysthymia were thought to have a character flaw that they could overcome with willpower. They were told to brighten up and be happy – as if they could change their mood by simply trying harder.

Double Depression

Double depression is the condition of dysthymia interspersed with episodes of major depression. These episodes can develop even though the person is already receiving treatment for dysthymia. At that point, the treatment will be reviewed and adjusted.

Seasonal Affective Disorder

Carol used to be outgoing and fun to be with. However, for the past three years she has hibernated in the winter. She feels exhausted after working eight hours. She drags herself home and naps in front of the television. When friends call her to go out, she doesn't have the energy. She feels unhappy and lonely but can't shake off the tiredness. Even when her friends beg her, she finds some excuse to avoid them; the grey skies and cold weather defeat her. As soon as the days begin to get longer in the spring, her energy returns. She doesn't know how many more years she can tolerate the 'winter blues'.

Carol has a condition called seasonal affective disorder (SAD). Certain individuals are very sensitive to the alterations of light and dark that come with the long nights and short days of winter. The condition improves with light therapy; see Chapter 6 for details.

Atypical Depression

Ratna had difficulty getting up in the morning. Her limbs felt like lead, and it often took her about two hours to get ready for the day. She had gained about twenty pounds, though she wasn't eating that much more, and she felt sluggish and heavy. She was ashamed about her weight gain and lack of motivation. She had started to avoid spending time with her friends and family because their remarks about her appearance hurt her.

Overeating, oversleeping, terrible fatigue, and heightened sensitivity to rejection are the core symptoms of atypical depression. Women are more frequently affected than men. This type of depression can change over time into one of the types described earlier. For example, someone like Ratna may develop the signs of a major depressive episode, but with retardation of movement, too much eating, and too much sleeping rather than symptoms such as agitation, not eating, and not sleeping.

Masked Depression (Somatization Disorder)

Depression is an illness that affects the whole body, not just the brain and mind. But in masked depression the physical symptoms are more prominent. You are less affected by emotional changes, such as sadness, hopelessness, and guilt, but are preoccupied with your physical distress. The regulatory functions of the body seem out of balance.

You may go to your family doctor complaining of vague but persistent physical symptoms. You worry about some serious undiscovered illness, such as cancer. You may experience bloating in your stomach, vomiting, pain, and nausea. You can feel diffuse backaches and headaches. You may complain of chest pain, dizziness, palpitations (rapid, irregular heartbeat), generalized weakness, difficulty swallowing, and memory loss. Your family doctor will investigate your various problems to rule out any underlying physical illness. When the depression is treated, any related physical symptoms should diminish or disappear.

Masked depression is more common in the elderly and in those cultures in which people are less likely to talk about their feelings. Young children who are depressed are also more likely to report physical rather than emotional symptoms.

Disorders Similar to Depression

Normal Bereavement

Your reaction to the death of a loved one can show many characteristics similar to depression. But you are not considered clinically depressed because the experience of grief, pervasive sadness, difficulty sleeping, emotional pain, and disengagement is universal. In normal bereavement there is less suicidal thinking, less slowed thinking, less slow moving, and less worry about past actions than in the disorder of depression.

A survivor may feel especially intense grief if the death is sudden and unexpected, if he or she feels blamed, or has difficulty expressing feelings, or is socially isolated. Only when someone develops more alarming and prolonged symptoms – such as guilt, agitation, and delusions – do we classify the person as depressed.

Chronic Fatigue Syndrome (CFS)

It's often difficult to distinguish between this syndrome and depression, because the symptoms can be similar. To further complicate matters, people with CFS can develop depression as well, because of the restrictions of the illness, and because some of the professionals they consult may minimize their distress. The syndrome itself is distinct from depression. The leaden heaviness of the limbs, the lack of energy after sleeping, and the inability to function – often accompanied by fibromyalgia (pain where muscles meet the bones) – are signs of this illness, but the exact cause of CFS is not known.

Post-Traumatic Stress Disorder

The complexities of this disorder became better understood after soldiers returned from Vietnam in the 1960s. The symptoms of some of the veterans were recognized as being common to people had been exposed to overwhelming trauma without adequate communal support. Survivors of previous wars or the Holocaust, and victims of childhood sexual abuse, showed the same pattern. This syndrome can be accompanied by depression but it has its own distinctive features – flashbacks, nightmares, and overwhelming fears provoked by seemingly innocuous stimuli that the person does not consciously connect with the original trauma.

Disorders Occurring with Depression

Personality Disorders

This large category of illnesses affects about 20 per cent of the population. Someone with a personality disorder has inappropriate, maladaptive responses to other people that can cause misunderstanding and dissension. Even after friends and family respond negatively, the person continues the irritating behaviours. For example, when Martin and Derek were discussing financial figures, Martin remarked, 'I don't understand how you're coming up with that number.' Derek, who has a personality disorder, took this as a personal criticism and lashed out in response: 'Do your own thinking from now on! I'll never suggest anything again!' His inappropriate reaction put an end to their meeting.

The characteristic patterns of personality disorders are thought to develop in childhood, because of the difficulty the child is having in adapting to the needs of a disturbed caregiver in order to stay attached to him or her. As an adult the person continues to use the same behaviours, but the behaviours evoke rejection rather than support.

People with personality disorders may become depressed when they fail to establish the relationships they crave. Some variants of depression can be misdiagnosed as a personality disorder. In particular, the irritability and withdrawal of dysthymia can be mistaken for symptoms of a personality disorder.

Panic Disorder

A panic attack is a sudden, intense fear that may be accompanied by a pounding heart, perspiration, trembling, a choking sensation, chest pain, nausea, dizziness, and fear of losing control or dying. These attacks can recur, and are absolutely terrifying. They can be controlled with medications or behaviour therapy and are often seen in people who suffer from depression.

Obsessive-Compulsive Disorder

Someone with an obsessive-compulsive disorder has recurrent distressing thoughts and impulses that cannot be shaken off. The person may also feel compelled to perform certain behaviours even though they don't make sense. If he or she does not carry out these behaviours, acute anxiety results. Again, symptoms of this disorder often occur among people with depression.

Schizophrenia

Schizophrenia is a severe chronic mental illness characterized by difficulties in all areas of functioning, and distortions in perception and reasoning. Twenty-five per cent of people with this disorder suffer from depression as well.

What Causes Depressive Illness?

No one knows exactly what causes a depressive episode. We do know that genetic makeup and events early in life predispose

Moods and humours

The ancient Greeks recognized that people had different natural temperaments, and both health and temperament were attributed to the balance of four liquids (called humours) in the body. If you had too much black bile you would be depressed and melancholic (melas is Greek for 'black'); an excess of yellow bile would make you irritable and choleric (khole means 'bile'); if white phlegm predominated you would be apathetic and phlegmatic (phlegma also means 'bile'); and if red blood prevailed, you would be optimistic and sanguine (sanguis is Latin for 'blood'). If only it were that simple!

people to develop depression. We also know that stressful life events can precipitate a depressive episode. Some physical illnesses and medications can increase the chances of developing such an episode. We are rapidly learning about the chemical changes that occur in the body when you develop one. All these factors, under the right circumstances, can lead to a depressive disorder.

Upsetting events happen to everyone at some time. Depression often develops when the event is connected with loss of some sort, such as death, divorce, financial losses, job loss, or loss of status. But some people may have characteristics that make them more likely to develop a depressive illness. Your genetic endowment, the quality of your early attachments, your temperament, your sex, and your personality style can all contribute. Even if you have characteristics that predispose you to depression, it will not develop every time there is a loss in your life. However, a depressive episode is six times more common within six months after a stressful life event than at other times.

Genetics

If you develop depression, there may be a history of depressive illness in your close blood relatives. When a parent is affected, a child has a much higher than average chance of developing the illness. When both parents are affected, a child has an even greater chance of being ill. If you have brothers or sisters with depressive disorder, you are two to four times more likely to develop the illness than if no relatives are affected. In identical twins, who have identical genes, if one twin develops the illness, the chance of the other also developing it is about 50 per cent. In fraternal twins, whose genes are no more similar than those of other siblings, there is a 25 to 33 per cent chance of the second twin also developing the illness. Adopted children develop depression at a rate influenced by their natural parents, not their adoptive parents. A number of different genes, in combination, predispose someone to depression.

Studies show that genetic inheritance plays a substantial part in the development of a depressive disorder. But even if you have the genetic makeup for depression, you will not necessarily develop the illness. If enough negative factors act on you, the illness will appear. With enough positive factors – such as good relationships, success at work, and a stable lifestyle – the illness will not develop, or will be easier to treat.

Early Attachment

If you lose a parent in childhood, by death or permanent separation, you have a higher risk of developing a depressive illness as an adult. Studies from ethology, the science of animal behaviour and its parallels in human behaviour, have shown that an infant forms an emotional attachment to its mother in order to survive. An infant rejected or abandoned by the mother may develop a severe depression. Many infants whose mothers died during World War Two in the carpet-bombing of London, and who were placed in austerely run orphanages, developed severe depressive illness. More recently, many infants in orphanages in Romania who received minimal physical care and affection were found to be severely depressed.

There is evidence that children who are rejected emotionally or harshly treated by their natural parents develop similar problems. Some studies show that decreased paternal care in childhood also leads to depression that responds poorly to treatment. Indeed, in some cases, a parent cannot provide the attachment to ensure a child's security because of life stresses or a depressive illness that the parent is going through while caring for the child.

Temperament

We are born with temperaments that stay with us throughout life. In early infancy, children's temperaments are characterized by their energy levels, sleeping patterns, eating patterns, and responsiveness to the environment. They can be easy and adaptable, slow to warm up, or difficult to handle. If the parent has difficulty matching the child's rhythm and temperament, problems can develop in their emotional attachment.

Sex

Major depressive disorder is twice as common in women as it is in men. Both hormone changes and social changes contribute to this difference. The reasons are discussed in detail in Chapter 9, 'Women and Depression'.

Personality

People who develop major depressive disorder are often conscientious, perfectionistic, and self-critical. They look to others for approval and acceptance. They also like to feel that everything is under control. Consequently, they can be thrown by the unpredictability of fate. How we behave doesn't guarantee good luck, but people who are prone to depression tend to blame themselves when things don't work out. They also feel very angry much of the time, but rarely express the anger directly.

Your personality can protect you against the development of depression, or promote its development. Four well-recognized characteristics are associated with the tendency toward depression.

- *Low self-esteem.* People with a negative outlook, with no abiding belief in their own worth, lack resilience and the ability to cope with adversity and solve problems.
- *Neuroticism.* When people are predisposed to recognize harm and danger in situations, they find life events overwhelming and difficult to change. Their thoughts are characterized by worry, emotionality, pessimism, and dissatisfaction.
- *Avoidance.* Some people withdraw from novel situations and see personal challenges as threats. They are shy, anxious, and depressed, and may use substances such as alcohol to dull painful feelings.
- *Impulsivity.* Some people have trouble moderating their

emotions, are quick to anger, seek novelty, and have difficulty waiting for rewards.

Social Support Network

The social world provides meaning, acceptance, and help for the stressed individual. The complexity, uncertainty, and rapid changes in our world put stress on all of us. A partner and children who love us, friends who care, and adequate food and shelter all help us deal with adversities.

A study in Nova Scotia, Canada, started years ago and still proceeding, shows that socially disintegrating communities have higher rates of depression. Socially disintegrating communities are defined as having social disruption with inadequate provisions for the poor, violence, a lack of community organization, inadequate education, and inadequate disease control. Another large study in the United States showed similar findings.

Single mothers living on social assistance with young children have an alarming rate of clinical depression. This group tends to be unsupported, isolated, and disadvantaged. Another study, in Britain, showed that married women whose marriages lacked intimacy, and who had no confiding relationship outside the home, were more likely to develop depression.

Because depressed people can be difficult to deal with at times, they may have less of the very support that would help them fight their depression.

Psychological Trauma

Depression – the illness – often follows the loss of a close friend or relative, or of something else very meaningful, such as a career or important possession. It is not the same as normal grieving. People tend to recover better from a personal loss such as a death than from an achievement loss such as being fired from a job, perhaps because there is less loss of self-esteem. In bereavement there are fewer thoughts of suicide, fewer worries about past actions, and less mental and physical slowness than in depression.

Freud thought that depression resulted when a person was unable to grieve adequately. Depressed people cannot allow themselves to express sadness because it's too painful. They are afraid of being destroyed by the intensity of their feelings. Instead, they avoid the grief by distracting themselves. But going through the painful feelings eventually helps us deal with our loss and move on. Someone who cannot grieve cannot accept the changes, but clings to the past with rage and anger. In grieving we feel rage and anger too, but in time we reach a stage of acceptance and resignation, even though we realize that life will never be the same. The depressed person who cannot go through grieving also cannot accept the permanent alterations in life.

Medical Disorders

HORMONAL DISORDERS

Hormones are messenger chemicals that travel through the bloodstream, communicating between the brain and the body to regulate systems or glands that need to be adjusted frequently. These glands may go out of balance when there are changes in the environment or the internal state of the individual. A feedback system between the glands and the brain acts to maintain the balance. Think of the operation of the thermostat on your furnace. When the temperature goes down, the thermostat signals the furnace to turn up the heat. When the house becomes too hot, the thermostat signals the furnace to stop producing heat. The thermostat is acting like the brain, and the signals are acting like hormones.

Several of these regulatory systems or glands can alter our emotions. The thyroid gland regulates our metabolism and is located in front of the throat. When the thyroid gland is too active, we call the illness hyperthyroidism. When the thyroid gland is underactive, we call that hypothyroidism. Depression can be a symptom of both illnesses.

The parathyroid is a very small gland that sits on the thyroid gland. This gland regulates calcium balance, which in turn regulates muscle firing. When this gland is overactive, the illness is called hyperparathyroidism. The person can experience depression as well as fatigue, nausea, vomiting, and excessive urination.

The adrenal glands, located on top of the kidneys, regulate our response to stress. In stressful situations, the level of cortisone, the hormone produced by the adrenal gland, increases. People with Addison's disease produce too little cortisone and can develop depression. People with Cushing's syndrome produce too much cortisone and can also develop depression. They also have an obese upper body, high blood pressure, and a round, red face. (Cushing's syndrome can also occur when someone is given cortisone or steroids as medication.)

The gonadal glands regulate our reproductive functions. Depression can occur in women when there is an imbalance of the gonadal hormones. This is discussed in more detail in Chapter 9.

The pancreas is a gland located behind the stomach that produces insulin, which regulates sugar metabolism. People who are diabetic produce too little insulin. Twenty-five per cent of people with diabetes develop depression. The direct cause is unknown.

The pituitary gland, located at the base of the brain, coordinates the feedback between all these glands and the brain. Interactions between the limbic system of the brain (which is concerned with automatic functions such as temperature and sleep regulation, as well as emotional reactions), the frontal lobe of the brain, and the pituitary gland can alter our emotions and cause depressive illness.

INFECTIONS

Viral illnesses often leave someone depressed after the acute illness is over. The reason is not clear, but the phenomenon is seen in influenza, viral pneumonia, viral hepatitis, infectious mononucleosis, and AIDS.

AUTOIMMUNE DISEASES

Rheumatoid arthritis and systemic lupus erythematosus are autoimmune diseases that affect many body systems – joints, skin, kidneys, and brain. The underlying problem is an allergic reaction to the body's own tissue. Depression is often one of the symptoms of these diseases.

NUTRITIONAL DEFICIENCIES

Decreased absorption of certain nutrients can show up as depression before other symptoms are present. Both vitamin B12 deficiency and folic acid deficiency can produce depressive illness before the blood counts show anaemia, the symptom that usually alerts the doctor to these deficiencies. The fact that brain changes causing depression may show up first, before the anaemia, has only recently been recognized.

NEUROLOGICAL ILLNESSES

Many neurological (brain and spinal-cord) illnesses are accompanied by depression that results directly from the illness, not from the person's distress at being ill. The illness affects the same parts of the brain that are thought to malfunction in depression. Multiple sclerosis, Parkinson's disease, brain injuries, epilepsy, strokes, and brain tumours can all have depression as part of the picture. In elderly people, it can be difficult to distinguish between the onset of a dementia (such as Alzheimer's disease) and a reversible, treatable depression.

HEART DISEASE

Depression and heart disease are related. Many factors that lead to heart disease, such as smoking, weight fluctuations, high cholesterol, and high blood pressure, are also increased in people with depression. A large study of the general population in the United States showed that people who were depressed at the time of the study had four times as many deaths in the next fifteen months as did those who were not depressed. Sixty-three per cent of these deaths were due to heart disease or stroke. Another study showed that 16 per cent of people are depressed after a heart attack, and that this group has five times as many deaths within the next six months as those who are not depressed.

Some people are depressed before and after heart surgery such as a bypass operation, opening the arteries, or a heart transplant. The rate of depression decreases if the person has emotionally involved and caring relatives, goes for cardiac rehabilitation, and sees a psychiatrist before and after the surgery.

METABOLIC ILLNESSES

Two very rare metabolic illnesses can also begin with depression – Wilson's disease and acute intermittent porphyria. Wilson's disease is an inherited disorder of copper metabolism that leads to a buildup of copper in the body, particularly in the liver, cornea, and brain. Porphyria is an inherited disease caused by lack of a blood enzyme, and symptoms include nausea, vomiting, constipation, muscle weakness, vision problems, and paralysis.

TUMOURS

Sometimes an underlying brain malignancy will first appear as depression, before the cancer itself is diagnosed.

Medications

Certain medications used to treat medical illnesses can cause depression as a side effect. If you develop depression after you start using blood pressure medication, many forms of steroid medications, anti-inflammatory drugs, and anti-cancer chemotherapy drugs, your doctor may consider the possibility that the depression is a side effect of the medication.

Substance Abuse

Some street drugs, such as amphetamines and cocaine, leave the individual depressed after both prolonged use and withdrawal, because they use up the chemicals that sustain a

---

Depression is a possible effect of:
- *cimetidine* – used for gastric reflux, gastric and duodenal ulcers
- *bromocriptine, levodopa, selegiline* – used for Parkinson's disease
- *atenolol, reserpine, doxazosin* – used for high blood pressure
- *lorazepam, alprazolam* – used for anxiety
- *dexamethasone, prednisone, hydrocortisone* – used for allergies, arthritis, and autoimmune diseases, among others
- *ibuprofen, diclofenac, indomethacin* – used for pain and inflammation
- *vincristine, methotrexate* – used for cancer

---

normal mood level to prolong the 'high' the user craves. Alcohol can also cause depression, after both short-term and long-term use. This can be a vicious circle, as people often begin using alcohol to combat depressed feelings. It can be difficult to know which began first, the depression or the alcohol abuse. As well, there is probably a genetic overlap between depression and alcoholism. Fifty per cent of alcoholics develop depression, and 25 per cent of people with major depressive disorder abuse alcohol at some point.

Diagnosis

The variety of these disorders illustrates the complexity of depression, and all its associated factors. At present we have no practical, reliable biological marker to distinguish the person who suffers from a depression serious enough to require treatment from the person who feels only mildly depressed and will recover with support and time. A doctor judges the difference by considering the person's physical health, symptoms, the cause of the problem and the age of onset, life events, and the history and family history. The presence of a number of symptoms such as depressed mood, guilt feelings, decreased interests and activities, increased nervousness, physical symptoms of anxiety, decreased energy, and suicidal thoughts all indicate a depressive illness. Doctors and patients hope that we will find simpler measures in the future, so treatment can begin earlier and needless suffering can be prevented.

3
Bipolar Disorders

Trevor, a mechanic who worked in his father's machine shop, was happily married but childless. He began acting quite strangely shortly after his brother had a son. He started to stay up late at night, working alone in his garage. He told his wife, Eunice, that he had invented a motor that could run on propane only, and he thought Ford would buy his invention. He became more and more talkative, with monologues far into the night that Eunice found exhausting. If she protested, he became irate, saying she didn't appreciate him. Then he withdrew all their savings from the bank, for a reason he refused to explain. Uncharacteristically, he berated Eunice for interfering in his life. He was physically much bigger, towering over her and shaking his fist at her.

Eunice called her father-in-law, who talked quietly to Trevor. Trevor then broke into tears, rocking back and forth and lamenting what a failure he was.

Trevor's father told Eunice that Trevor's aunt had suffered from bipolar I, also known as manic-depressive illness. They took Trevor to the local hospital and he agreed to be admitted. After he had calmed down, he said he had felt great, as if his ideas were brilliant. He needed little sleep and his thoughts raced. He said that he had never felt so wonderful in his life, but that he also felt he was on a roller coaster that he couldn't get off.

Bipolar illness appears to be less common than depressive disorders, affecting only 2 per cent of the population at any given time. However, this figure is probably an underestimate, as people who have bipolar illness are frequently not aware of being ill, even if their close relatives know. The illness is chronic and recurrent, interfering with the person's ability to lead a productive and satisfying life. Fortunately, treatment can be very effective.

Many highly creative people have been affected with bipolar disorder. Winston Churchill could be amazingly productive when hypomanic, but totally incapacitated when his 'black dogs' of depression took over. (Hypomania refers to an elated mood and excessive energy that are out of keeping with the circumstances but do not involve delusions or hallucinations.) The illness could be traced back four or more generations in Churchill's family. His father, Randolph, was notorious for excessive behaviours, sometimes brilliant, sometimes silly. His ancestor the first Duke of Marlborough, who waged wars in the time of Queen Anne, could be a brilliant strategist, and then become inactive for long periods.

Kate Millett, a prolific feminist writer, describes her bouts of bipolar illness in *The Loony-Bin Trip*. She talks about the stigma, the embarrassment, and her attempts to find the help she needed. At one point, on a holiday far from friends and help, she was unceremoniously committed to the chronic ward of an Irish mental hospital.

Kay Redfield Jamison is a professor of psychiatry at Johns Hopkins University in Maryland, USA. Early in her career she suffered severe bouts of mania and depression. She has helped to reduce the stigma of the illness by talking publicly about her experiences and writing about them. A brave account of her illness can be found in her book *An Unquiet Mind*.

Everyone's moods fluctuate over time, usually in response to good or bad events. Once the upsetting or exciting events are over, our mood returns to a level neither too sad nor too excited. If you suffer from bipolar illness, however, your moods are greatly exaggerated. You swing widely between elation and despair. You may not be aware of how disproportionate your responses are to the events that triggered them; they make perfect sense to you. Sometimes there are no particular triggering events, but you read profound meaning into minor coincidences. When you enter a manic phase, your mood starts to rise and your elation and energy become so excessive that, often within a few days, you lose control and judgement. You seem to have lost the ability to come down to a base line or 'normal' level of mood. Then your mood reverses, just as excessively. A woman who has suffered from bipolar disorder since her teens used to leave her doctor a phone message saying, 'I started into a depression at two-thirty Wednesday afternoon.' Although the doctor was sceptical of her precision at first, her predictions turned out to be surprisingly accurate.

Bipolar illness begins at an earlier age than depressive illness – usually in the late teens – and is often confused with schizophrenia in adolescents, because the manic phases can appear quite bizarre, with delusions and hallucinations. The illness seems to be starting at younger and younger ages. Sometimes young children diagnosed as having attention deficit and hyperactivity disorder are found to be in the early stages of a bipolar illness. Bipolar disorder occurs in all ethnic and cultural communities.

Bipolar disorders cause major disruptions in family functioning. Separation and divorce are common. Denial is pervasive; people deny problems, sadness, the pain of loss, and the need for others when they are in a manic phase. In a depressed phase, they are incapacitated and unable to function.

Bipolar I

Bipolar I illness is characterized by alternating, recurrent episodes of mania and depression. It can be diagnosed after just one episode of mania has occurred. While a depressive episode appears identical to the major depressive episode described in the last chapter, a manic episode shows a distinctive period of abnormally elevated mood lasting a week or more. The heightened intensity of emotion seems out of sync with the events in the person's life. Usually the mood is joyful, but it can quickly change to irritability and anger. The person may talk ceaselessly and not wait for a response from other people; ideas follow each other rapidly. Sometimes the sequence of thoughts makes little sense, but at other times the person may be witty and infectiously funny. He or she lacks good judgement, feeling cleverer and more talented than everyone else, and not understanding why anyone would be alarmed by his or her grandiose plans. The person sleeps little or not at all, and may spend large amounts of money, be sexually promiscuous, or insult people indiscriminately.

When is mania not mania?

Symptoms of several physical illnesses – such as hyperthyroidism (overactive thyroid gland), systemic lupus erythematosus, brain tumours, or epilepsy – or even head injuries can be mistaken for the mania of bipolar disorder. Drug and alcohol abuse and steroid medications can also cause symptoms that resemble mania. A thorough review of the person's medical history and a physical examination, including appropriate laboratory tests, will distinguish these conditions.

Relatives and friends become exhausted and exasperated. The doctor may recommend hospitalization for someone who seems to be 'a danger to himself or others'. If the person refuses hospitalization, wondering why anybody wants to interfere when he or she is feeling so good, involuntary hospitalization can be arranged for a specified period of time. How the decision is made is discussed in detail in Chapter 11.

Bipolar II

Angie was a very sociable, gregarious woman who attracted friends initially but often wore them out with her exuberance and constant nattering. She was involved in many volunteer organizations and seemed to know everyone in her neighbourhood. Her husband and children were often left without any dinner while Angie was busy talking on the neighbour's front step. Sometimes she couldn't seem to slow down enough to listen to her family. She was likeable but exhausting to be around. She never seemed able to plan ahead; the house was always in a mess, things got started but never finished, the children's lunches were never ready. When Angie took a part-time job at the local chemist's, the customers seemed to like her, but the manager finally had to ask her to leave because she was too distractible and chaotic.

Angie has a milder form of bipolar disorder called bipolar II, characterized by alternating periods of major depression and hypomanic episodes. Hypomanic episodes are less disruptive than manic episodes, and the person doesn't lose touch with reality. However, social and occupational functioning are impaired. If you have this disorder you are in overdrive. You sleep little, and you can be reactive and intrusive with other people; they like you at first but quickly become exhausted and irritated by your excessive energy. You have little awareness or empathy for other people, although you mean well. You speak rapidly and change topics frequently. But you show no signs of psychosis, and you are not out of touch with your surroundings.

Rapid Cycling Disorder

A variant of both these disorders is rapid cycling disorder. If you have more than four episodes of a bipolar mood disorder in one year, you have a rapid cycling disorder. Your mood disorder can be manic, hypomanic, depressive, or mixed in character. (A mixed episode has features of both mania and depression.) You never quite achieve a normal mood level. This condition occurs in 70 per cent of women and 20 per cent of men with bipolar disease. There is also another variant called ultrarapid cycling disorder.

Cyclothymia

Eddie, a thirty-five-year-old salesman, came to see his family doctor because 'I keep making a mess of things at work and with the women in my life.' He starts a new job or new relationship enthusiastically and people tend to like him at first, but as soon as the newness wears off Eddie begins to lose heart, stays in bed longer in the morning, doesn't show up for appointments, and is generally unreliable, so that bosses and girlfriends become exasperated with his apologies and his promises to do better. Yet Eddie is a bright and creative man when he's doing well, and can usually produce good work when he's 'on'. He's also charming and fun to be with, and quite warm, so he is sought after by females when he's 'on'. He's had this behaviour pattern since his teens. He was unable to finish university and never stayed long enough at a job to get past entry-level salary.

Eddie's father suffers from bipolar disorder, and has been hospitalized two or three times for depression. Once, when he was feeling good, he used the family savings to buy into a business that soon went bankrupt. The marriage almost ended at that point. Eddie's father has now been prescribed lithium and is doing much better. But the father's brother killed himself when he was twenty-two, and Eddie's paternal grandfather was a moody, depressed man who was a heavy drinker.

Eddie was affable and talkative when he went to his doctor, and did not appear distressed. But he was worried about his behaviour patterns, and wondered if he might have an illness similar to his father's.

Eddie is suffering from cyclothymic disorder. This means that he has had constant fluctuations in mood, with few periods of normal mood, for at least two years. His fluctuations are not severe enough to impair his functioning, but his constant shifts in mood make it difficult to maintain stable relations at work or personally.

About 50 per cent of people diagnosed with cyclothymic disorder have a history of substance abuse. The illness usually begins in late adolescence, and it's lifelong. However, it responds to treatment.

What Causes Bipolar Illness?

As with depressive illness, we aren't sure exactly what causes bipolar illness. The causes seem to differ somewhat from those listed for depressive disorders; external upsetting events are not as likely to precipitate an episode. Someone with a bipolar disorder almost always has a close relative who has a variant of the disorder. However, the incidence of bipolar illness is much lower than that of depressive illness. The chance of developing a bipolar illness over a lifetime is estimated to be between 0.6 and 0.9 per cent, although this too may be an underestimate. The chance of developing a major depressive disorder over a lifetime ranges from 2 to 12 per cent for men and from 5 to 26 per cent for women, depending on the study.

Genetics

The risk of inheriting a form of bipolar illness is higher than the risk of inheriting a depressive disorder. It's likely that defects in several genes work together to cause the illness. When one identical twin develops the illness, the other also develops it in 60 per cent of cases. If one fraternal twin develops it, the other will develop it in 30 per cent of cases. If a parent has a bipolar illness, a child has a higher chance of developing the illness. As in depressive disorder, the illness occurs whether or not the child is raised with the natural parents, so it seems to be caused by a genetic similarity rather than by the family environment, as has been shown by the adoption studies. Again, the genetic predisposition does not always cause the illness. There are other possible causes as well.

Sex

Men and women are affected equally in bipolar illness. However, about 70 per cent of women with bipolar illness have rapid cycling disorder, compared to 20 per cent among men. Women also have more bipolar II disorders than men. The diagnosis of bipolar II – sometimes referred to as soft bipolarity – can be missed.

Temperament

The people who seem most prone to develop bipolar illness are those who have an outgoing temperament. They are responsive to other people, and their enthusiasm and sense of fun can be very engaging. They can be carefree, sociable, and highly energetic. Many people with bipolar illness are also creative and artistic, and many work as artists and performers.

4
Getting Help

Now that you've had a chance to find out what depression looks like, and to consider whether you or a family member may be affected, let's look at possible ways of managing the disorder.

Many treatments and therapists are available. You'll have to decide what type of approach suits you best. Often this depends on where you live and, if you have health insurance, what type of treatment your insurance covers. A good place to start is probably with your general practitioner. He or she has a medical degree, can prescribe drugs, can investigate other possible causes for your symptoms and can refer you to local services. In urban centres, help may be available from the mental health clinic outpatient department of your local hospital. If you make an appointment, you may be seen in a relatively short time. You can be referred to a psychiatrist by your general practitioner, to be seen in his or her office. But resources are often limited, and few of these services are readily available outside of urban centres. In the UK, these

Who does psychotherapy?

Psychiatrists are often in short supply, particularly in smaller communities. Their waiting lists vary considerably but can be as long as three to four months. A family doctor may have had additional training in psychotherapy and can prescribe medications as well. Registered psychologists and social workers are also trained in psychotherapy but they can't prescribe drugs. Often, a patient receives psychotherapy from one person and has medications prescribed by another. Some of these professional services may not be covered by private insurance plans.

services are all covered by the NHS, however, if you have health insurance most companies provide the option of receiving treatment from private psychiatric hospitals and therapy services (according to their individual criteria).

Once you have made an initial contact, other reasons for the depression have to be considered. After a thorough medical checkup has been done, and it's been established that the depression doesn't seem related to a physical cause, you will want to find a therapist you can work with. Even if the initial recommendation is primarily for medication, such as antidepressants or mood stabilizers, you will need someone you can discuss your concerns and fears with, or you may end up stopping the medication and abandoning treatment. Choosing a therapist also involves finding someone you like and are comfortable talking to about private problems. If you feel judged or censored or talked down to, find someone else. If you feel the therapist is uninterested or bored, think twice, but remember that some of these feelings may be sorted out if you talk to the therapist. It's possible that you are misjudging the therapist. If you have felt overlooked and slighted by people in the past, you may expect this reaction now even when it's not there. You will also want to assess how honest the therapist is in telling you about his or her own reactions. Before you share many intimate details about your life with this person, you need to feel that he or she is trustworthy and competent. Ask around. If possible, start by considering several therapists, and meet with them to see if they are a good fit. If you hear positive comments about the same therapist from two or three different sources, that therapist is probably a good choice.

Prepare yourself for the fact that treatment takes time. There will be difficult and discouraging stages, and it's important not to jump ship hastily, thinking that there is better help elsewhere. Try to work things out with the therapist you are already with, and don't be afraid to talk about the problem. If you feel disrespected or otherwise uncomfortable, say so. This is all good practice in becoming more direct in your feelings. You may also find that, as a result of this openness and honesty, you develop a deeper and more productive relationship with your therapist that can enrich other relationships in your life.

Taking Care of Yourself

The type of treatment recommended depends on the severity of the depression, but there are some general rules for self-help that are simply common sense. If you are mildly depressed, it's best to keep as active as you can. Maintain regular habits, if possible. Try to maintain your sleep patterns, eat regular healthy meals, cut down on caffeine and alcohol, go for walks, and get up, showered, and dressed every morning. In this way, you may be able to prevent the depression from spiralling downward. (This is much easier said than done, as anyone who has been there will tell you.) Talk to friends and family, join self-help groups, or join interest groups. Try choosing activities that provide pleasure. Expect less from yourself, and realize that it is perfectly acceptable to say 'No' or 'I don't know how'.

You also have to decrease stresses in your life, realizing that there are situations and events you can't control or change. It may help to use coping statements such as 'I am a capable person', or 'I've managed to get through tough times before and I can do it this time', or 'Not everyone has to approve of what I do'. You can even say them out loud.

Marcia, aged twenty-four, and her brother, Adam, at fifteen, had lost their parents in a motor accident. At first, Adam moved in with their uncle and aunt. After a few weeks, however, he began stealing from his aunt and refusing to attend school. Marcia, who was working in an office and living in her own flat, was asked to take over. She felt obligated to take care of Adam until he finished secondary school, so she moved to a two-bedroom flat. She also arranged for Adam to speak to a counsellor at an adolescent community treatment centre. Adam continued to play truant and refused to attend therapy sessions, so the counsellor discharged him and the school suspended him. He began stealing from Marcia, and refused to tell her where he was in the evenings. He slept until noon and left dirty dishes around the flat.

Marcia felt that, if she could only convince him of her love and devotion, he would start behaving himself. She became more and more depressed at her failure. Her boss said her work was slipping, and suggested she talk to the company counsellor.

The counsellor listened carefully to Marcia's story, and noted how sad and drawn she looked. The counsellor then saw Adam and Marcia together. Adam said how furious he was about their parents' death, and said that he felt Marcia owed him extra attention. The counsellor explained that while all this was painful for Adam, Marcia could not fill the emptiness, and arranged for Adam to be admitted to a home for troubled adolescents so that he could work on his difficulties. Marcia reluctantly agreed.

Marcia continued to support Adam on her days off. She started to feel better, and her work improved. Adam was finally able to mourn the loss of his parents, and give up the hope that he could bring them back.

When Is Professional Help Necessary?

You need professional help immediately if you are thinking actively about suicide. You also need professional help if you have more than three of the following symptoms:

- depressed mood
- guilt feelings
- loss of interest and pleasure
- tension, nervousness
- physical symptoms of anxiety
- low energy level

If the depression has not let up after two or more weeks, if you are losing weight, if you are having difficulty sleeping – particularly if you wake early in the morning in an agitated state and can't get back to sleep – you will not get better without help. If the depressive symptoms are this severe, you will need antidepressant medication. You will have difficulty focusing on psychotherapy unless you feel better. Therapy is hard work.

Recently, early and adequate treatment with anti-depressants has been recommended to eliminate the above symptoms of depression in most cases. This minimizes the number of recurrences, and the illness is less likely to become chronic. Psychotherapy alone is usually not enough.

Or you may have the opposite symptoms – you may sleep and eat excessively, may be unable to keep up with your work or home schedules, and may have little interest in pleasures you used to enjoy. Again, you need help. If you are experiencing intense anxiety, guilt you can't shake, or you are isolating yourself from friends and colleagues, consult a doctor or a counsellor. Talking to a therapist alone is not the solution here. You will need to start taking an antidepressant before you are able to use therapeutic help. Don't be embar-rassed to tell family and friends that you are going through a rough period and need extra support.

Sometimes, depression can become so severe that you feel flat, numb, and cut off from any feelings. The world seems black and awful, you feel miserable and are afraid you are going crazy. You may see suicide as a possible solution. You may develop psychotic symptoms such as delusions, fixed ideas with no basis in reality – you may be convinced that you have a terminal illness, or that you have committed a terrible sin. You may experience hallucinations, hearing voices condemning you. You may feel deeply agitated and unable to keep still.

This is a very serious condition and you need help immedi-ately. Let someone you can depend on know how bad you feel, and ask for help. You can go to the local A & E department, where there is a psychiatrist on call. Sometimes local hospitals have a crisis unit with staff specially trained to evaluate the severity of a condition like yours. You will certainly need to be started on medication and seen regularly. Voluntary admission to hospital may be suggested.

Knowledge can help you get the support you need. There are lots of resources available, but tapping into help that works for you is important. Sometimes, when you're depressed, you feel hopeless, as if nothing will change. This is not true. Time and care will make you feel better. To get the right care, you can use the same strategies you would use if you needed a good financial advisor or a good music teacher. Assess credentials, find out what to look for by reading or through the Internet, choose someone you like and 'click' with, and continue to do your homework, getting counselling, taking medication, using self-help strategies – whatever is right for you.

5
Psychosocial Therapies

Psychosocial therapies include all the 'talking therapies'. They can be very helpful for milder forms of depression. We can divide them into three major groups:

- cognitive behavioural
- interpersonal
- short-term psychodynamic

In day-to-day practice, most therapists use a combination of many types of therapy. Both the therapist and you are active – exchanging observations, ideas, and feelings in a comfortable private place. You are free to talk about what you like, while the therapist listens and asks questions in order to understand the issues. The old stereotype of the bearded analyst staring and saying nothing, like someone out of a Punch cartoon, has essentially gone the way of the horse and buggy.

The different types of therapy have common character-istics. In the first stage of therapy, a respectful and empathic relationship, sometimes referred to as a 'working alliance', develops between you and the therapist. The therapist listens carefully to how you define and understand your difficulties, deciphering when the problems started, how they are affecting you now, what makes you feel better and what worse, and what sort of changes might help. How does this differ from what a good friend or partner can offer? For one thing, your choices don't affect the therapist's own life. For another, everything you tell the therapist is held in confidence. The therapist has no set ideas about what is best for you. He or she will do more than try to cheer you up. Both of you work on clarifying the problem, how you are affected by it, and how you can act in your best interests with minimum negative consequences for your relatives and friends.

The relief in having a safe place to talk to someone who is actively trying to understand and make sense of your experience, without judging you, can be healing in itself. When differences arise between you and the therapist, you can talk about the conflict openly, not sweep it under the table as you might in social situations. This flexibility helps you explore different viewpoints without always having to decide on a right or wrong answer. It is also very gratifying to be given someone's complete attention and interest for an uninterrupted hour. Usually the sessions are once or twice a week for approximately twelve to twenty weeks.

It is useful to combine drug therapy with psychotherapy. Thoughts and feelings and chemical changes in the brain influence each other. When we change the way we think and feel, we change what is happening chemically in the brain. When we change the chemical balance in the brain with drugs, we change how we think and feel. That's why drugs

What are all these different therapies?

Psychotherapy is the treatment of people with emotional problems, primarily through talking. By exploring the patient's problems, the therapist helps the person change distressing thoughts, feelings, and behaviour. Psychotherapy can be done *individually*, or in a *group* of people, or with the whole *family*. *Short-term therapy* may involve anything from one to twenty sessions, depending on the patient's needs or the limits imposed by insurers.

Psychoanalytic theory, originated by Sigmund Freud, is based on an understanding of human behaviour accumulated by generations of analysts in the course of their work.

Psychoanalysis is the classic pattern of one-hour treatment four or five days a week over several years. By sharing childhood experiences, dreams, reflections, and feelings with the therapist, the patient gains understanding and the ability to change as he or she wishes.

Psychodynamic therapy is based on psychoanalytic theory. *Psychoanalytically* based psychotherapy has been modified to meet time and financial constraints.

Psychosocial therapy deals with emotional problems that result partly from social interactions.

Psychoeducational therapy includes education about the disorder, to help the person deal with it.

Cognitive behavioural therapy is developed from the principles of learning theory, and examines the ways automatic patterns of thinking shape our behaviour.

Interpersonal therapy focuses on the 'here and now': the way someone copes with loss in the current social environment.

and psychotherapy can work together, reinforcing each other.

At some point, you may have to deal with sadness and anger over a permanent change in your life that you can't control. Such adjustments can be very painful. Perhaps you have lost someone you love, or the future you had hoped for. Losses like this can leave anyone disappointed and angry, but if you are predisposed to develop depression, you may be convinced that the loss is entirely your fault, and that you are helpless and incapable of controlling what happens to you. If you are unable to get past this guilt and self-blame, you are very likely to become depressed. When you are able to voice your grief and rage without being silenced, your feelings are validated – they are accepted as reasonable and understandable. You can then eventually move past the loss, taking joy in life as it now is.

Early in treatment, your therapist should give you an explanation of what he or she sees happening to you and what can be done about it. This should be in clear language; if you don't understand any of it, say so. The therapist will be aware of any embarrassment you feel about coming for help, and needs to be aware of your doubts about your treatment. You may have had bad experiences in the past with caregivers, such as parents, teachers, and doctors, that make you sceptical about receiving care. Even one bad experience can make you wary and uncomfortable.

Tyrell had once been assessed in a large auditorium with medical students watching. He had been humiliated and unable to say a coherent word. Later, the doctor asked his wife what it was like to live with someone who was so seriously ill. Needless to say, it took months before Tyrell overcame this experience and managed to see another therapist!

The therapist can only build up your sense of trust by being consistent and caring over time. In short-term therapy, you usually contract with a therapist to work on your difficulties for some ten to twelve weekly sessions of about an hour each. During that time you may discuss issues that are bothering you currently, what it is about you that makes these issues particularly disruptive, where those feelings originated, and how they might be altered. As you go through the therapy, you begin to notice that certain patterns recur between you and the people you interact with in the present, between you and your therapist, and between you and important people in your past. Once the patterns are identified, they can be modified. You may also come to understand how your family or other caregivers pass on to you the stresses or depressions they themselves are burdened by. Through understanding, you can use behaviours that work rather than behaviours from the past that hinder your present relationships.

Types of Therapists

Various types of therapists are available. National licensing bodies regulate the qualifications, competence, and ethical conduct of the following practitioners.

- A psychiatrist is a medical doctor who has several years' further training in psychiatry. Psychiatrists are trained to conduct psychotherapy, to prescribe medication, and to diagnose medical illnesses that may cause psychiatric disorders.
- Family doctors may also do psychotherapy, as well as diagnosing medical causes of depression and prescribing drugs. Any additional training in psychotherapy after medical school is left to their discretion.
- A clinical psychologist has been trained in psychological theory and psychotherapy skills under the supervision of practising psychologists at a university.
- A community psychiatric nurse is a registered nurse who works in the community providing practical advice,

ongoing support with problems, supervises medication, gives injections and helps with supportive counselling.
- Occupational therapists are trained to help depressed clients develop the abilities they need for independent living in order to become active and involved in society once more. These can include occupational and employment-related skills training and creative activities such as art.

Note that psychologists, nurses and occupational therapists are not physicians, and are not permitted to prescribe medication.

Many good training programmes teach skills in different types of psychotherapy and offer diplomas specifying the skills learned. But don't assume that a self-described expert has acceptable training. Inquire about the person's schooling, and ask to see a list of qualifications.

Employee Assistance Programs (EAP) and Extended Health Insurance Plans often cover the cost of therapy services, but they usually specify the category of therapist they will pay for and the length of treatment. Feel free to ask for all the information you need to make an informed decision, as a patient and as a consumer. You can also call the licensing body to check the person's credentials.

Your choice of therapist ultimately depends on whether you like the person and feel comfortable confiding in him or her – and whether you are satisfied that the therapist is competent and cares about you. From your point of view, your comfort and confidence in the therapist are paramount. You want to feel better but you simply don't have the resources to make it happen. Your therapist can help you learn more about depression, and about how to lessen its effects.

Cognitive Behavioural Therapy

Cognitive behavioural therapy, or CBT, is based on the principles of learning theory. If you are prone to depression, you tend to think globally and see catastrophes everywhere. Some common distortions in thinking are *selective abstraction* – noticing only the worst details; *overgeneralization* – seeing disaster everywhere from a single event; *all-or-nothing thinking* – magnifying bad events, and minimizing good events; *personalization* – attributing blame to yourself for neutral events; and *extremes of idealization and devaluation* of people important in your life – seeing them as either entirely benevolent and kind, or entirely bad and malicious.

Kareena would always see herself as falling short because she couldn't meet her expectations at work. Whenever she was asked specifically what she needed to do to feel satisfied with herself, she would overgeneralize, and answer that she had 'masses' of reports to write, 'masses' of washing to do, 'masses' of people to call. She had to work with her therapist to translate her 'masses' into more realistic, manageable obligations.

Similarly, Sarah told her friend Ann that she felt she needed less advice and direction from her, and Ann became angry; she felt she had simply been helping. When Sarah reported this incident to her therapist, she insisted that Ann would never forgive her – even though they had been friends since secondary school, and had always enjoyed being together. Sarah was sure she'd lost her friend forever. This is an example of 'all or nothing' thinking, which is usually negative.

The 'learned helplessness' theory of depression, developed

by Martin Seligman, a psychologist at the University of Pennsylvania in the United States, suggests how helpless or hopeless depressive behaviour can begin in humans. Behaviour in experimental animals sometimes parallels human behaviour. Rats were placed on an electric grid that administered a shock to them. They were able to escape the shock by jumping to a part of the grid that was shock-free. They quickly learned to avoid the shock. However, some rats were first placed on a grid with no means of escaping the shock, no matter what they did. After several trials there, they were placed on the grid that allowed them to escape. But these rats never tried to escape the shock, though all they had to do was jump to the other side of the grid. Seligman speculates that something similar may happen to humans who are repeatedly exposed to failure; they lose heart and can no longer muster the strategies to escape their situation.

Dr Aaron Beck, an American psychiatrist and psychoanalyst who originated CBT, described the 'negative cognitive triad' of depression. You have a negative view of yourself, of the world (including other people), and of the future. You see yourself as defective, deprived or inadequate. You may feel that 'Everyone would be happier if I were dead.' You may tend to interpret all external events as negative, and you predict disasters and failures in the future. The therapist can deal with the defences you put up in your resistance to getting well, such as reluctance to reveal your thoughts and feelings, insistence on managing alone, or – paradoxically – expectation that the therapist should do all the work. You will begin to identify the thoughts that develop automatically whenever you are in stressful situations; these thoughts are often based on false premises, and new, more adaptive responses can be learned.

John visited the university health service at the beginning of April. He was in the second year of an honours BA in economics, but he was fearful that he wouldn't do well on his upcoming exams. When questioned further, he also said that he had lost some weight, was not interested in going out with his friends, and was sleeping poorly. The counsellor began to see John weekly, to treat his depression with cognitive therapy. John wrote down what he was feeling when he was stressed and what he did about it, conscientiously recording his reactions and his accompanying thoughts. Eventually, he and the counsellor began to notice a pattern. Whenever John failed to achieve what he had set out to do, he berated himself for being a no-hoper and a failure, and told himself that he would never achieve anything worthwhile. At that point he would stop working. Together, John and his counsellor began to reframe his thoughts so that he didn't give up each time he reached an impasse. John practised these new skills until he was able to complete what he had set out to do. He reached a point where he felt confident about passing his exams, and his depressive symptoms improved.

In cognitive behavioural therapy, the therapist does not act as an expert and suggest behaviours to you; this simply doesn't work. Instead, through reflection, clarification, and questioning of your basic assumptions, the therapist tries to help you develop alternative ways of thinking, so that you can apply these to finding new, more positive ways of seeing yourself, others and the world.

Interpersonal Therapy

Interpersonal therapy is a short-term, focused form of therapy that concentrates on your interpersonal problems – that is, the problems you are having in dealing with other people in the here and now. Education and practical advice about depressive illness are included as part of the therapy. In many situations, interpersonal struggles and poor social interactions contribute to depression. An interpersonal therapist suggests how you might change the way you behave with others in order to receive the social support and understanding you need.

Major social changes in your life are the main focus of this therapy, as they are thought to trigger depression if you are vulnerable. Grief and significant loss – whether through death, divorce, job loss or something else – are discussed. Periods of role transition, such as retirement from work or children leaving home, are also times of increased stress. Role disputes such as conflicts at work or in your marriage can lead to a drop in self-esteem and depression. One area that is more of a lifelong difficulty is poor interpersonal skills, so that you are never able to develop intimate and sustaining relationships. The therapist will explore these four areas of difficulty – grief and loss, role transition, role disputes and interpersonal skills – and together you can find alternate and more adaptable ways of managing.

As mentioned before, most therapists use parts of all types of therapy, and other techniques as well, to help you change. Both CBT and interpersonal therapy have been shown, in well-designed research studies, to improve depression. Both are equally effective, and both can be used for group therapy as well as one-on-one therapy.

Short-Term Psychodynamic Psychotherapies

Yvonne had never felt very confident. When she was a child, her older brother, Leo, excelled at school and at sports. He was also good-looking and charming, so he had many friends. Both parents, particularly the father, doted on Leo and constantly pointed out his accomplishments to anyone who would listen.

Yvonne was quiet and not as outgoing. She loved Leo but often felt unloved and unwanted. She coped with her feelings by spending most of her day at school or at friends' houses. This worked until she tried to go to university but was not accepted. She had wanted to be a lawyer like her father, but this goal now seemed out of reach.

Yvonne became less and less confident, and more and more listless and uninterested in going out and doing anything.

Her family doctor suggested that Yvonne see a psychiatrist. The parents were sceptical but finally agreed. The psychiatrist felt that Yvonne's depression and lack of interest were related to her feelings of inadequacy throughout childhood. He encouraged her to work on resolving those feelings, and assured her that she was a valuable and likable person, even though she was not as extroverted as her brother.

Psychodynamic therapies can treat depression, but they are not for depression alone. The therapist works from theories based on psychoanalytic principles originally developed by Sigmund Freud, and altered since then by other psychoanalysts, based on their experience with patients. The therapist assumes that events from your past are affecting the way you see and act in the present, although you may not be fully aware of how you are being affected. The experiences are buried in your unconscious mind, and the goal of this therapy is to remember and unravel the experiences and the ways they are now influencing you. When you become more aware of how the past affects you, you will be better able to decide how you want to live and act now.

People who are prone to depression often live their lives for some 'dominant other'. They feel that if they can only be what the more powerful person wants them to be, they'll gain love and care. When they don't receive that love and care, depression results; they feel that they are a failure because they can't satisfy the other person. However, their disappointment is based on a false premise. We all have to live for ourselves. When we become comfortable with our own feelings, good and bad, we are free to live lives that are truly our own.

In Freud's classic 1917 paper 'Mourning and Melancholia', he compared depression to grief. Although the depressed person does not actually lose a loved person, as in bereavement, he does lose the emotional connection with the loved person. The individual blames himself, experiencing guilt, shame, lowered self-esteem and 'anger turned inward'. He is angry and disappointed in the loved one, but cannot express his rage, for fear of being further rejected by the person whose emotional support he feels is necessary for his survival. The short-term psychoanalytic therapist works from these premises when seeing you.

Combining Psychotherapy and Medication

As mentioned in Chapter 4, studies have shown that if you are suffering from the symptoms of depression – depressed mood, guilt feelings, loss of interest and pleasure, tension and nervousness, physical symptoms of anxiety, low energy level, and/or suicidal thoughts – treating your first episode with antidepressants until the symptoms are gone changes the course of the illness and decreases the number of recurrences. Psychotherapy can enhance the action of the antidepressants, and can also teach you new coping strategies. The primary goal of treatment is to leave you with no residual symptoms of depression, so that the illness won't become more severe over time. One of the most difficult paradoxes in treating depression is that when people are most depressed, they are least likely to be aware of how impaired they are. They may be reluctant to take medication even though it can be a life-saver. At this point, the doctor and family must be persistent about the need for medication, but they must also acknowledge the person's fears about what is happening, and whether the illness can be safely treated. Usually, the therapist can combine a number of approaches, including education, the talking therapies and medication when it's indicated.

Family-Focused Therapy

When someone in a family develops depression, the rest of the family usually starts out feeling protective and compassionate, and tries to instill hope. But they can become discouraged when their efforts don't produce any reward.

Meanwhile, the depressed person is full of helpless and horrible feelings, which in turn evoke a tremendous sense of guilt and powerlessness in those who are trying to help. This guilt can be paralyzing, as family members feel they have somehow caused the illness. Everyone becomes angry and resentful, but tries to hide these shameful feelings.

The advantage of family therapy is that the whole family can talk about these painful feelings together. The frustration diminishes when other family members realize that they can't control or change the illness, any more than the depressed person can. With this understanding, they can be involved and helpful without the anguish of guilt and anger, and they can be much more realistic about what they can and cannot do.

Families are often ashamed of their relative's illness, and they may try to conceal it from friends and neighbours because they are afraid of gossip and prejudice. Since family therapy lessens their feeling of responsibility for the illness, it helps relieve this burden of secrecy and embarrassment. As well, it can lead to a more open relationship between family members, so that there is less risk of painful misunderstandings that might cause relatives to withdraw from each other.

Cognitive Styles That Make Depression Worse

Perfectionistic traits sometimes make it hard for depressed people to accept and use the help being offered to them; to their minds, this help never seems quite good enough or accurate enough. One woman whose life was hampered by her obsessive traits would never take her therapist's explanation of a medication at face value. She would consult friends in the mental health field, and search out professional bibliographies until she understood every aspect of the treatment. She would fuss over the dosage and worry about even the most minor and unlikely side effect.

If you try to find an explanation for absolutely everything in life, you can exhaust yourself by thinking in circles, ruminating over where the illness developed, and what negative traits in you or others have contributed to it. This accounting can become time-consuming and detrimental, and in some situations it may even hinder your recovery.

Lifelong patterns of suppressing anger, silencing yourself, and preserving relationships by giving in to others may perpetuate your depressive illness. If you continue in your old patterns, you may also erupt in 'anger attacks' that can be hurtful to those around you and jeopardize the relationships you value. Learning to deal directly with the people you are close to, by stating what you feel and what you want to change, can be frightening at first but exhilarating in the long run. Moreover, it is easier on the people around you, as it allows them to talk openly about difficulties and conflicts that they feel.

Psychosocial Therapy for Bipolar Illness

Bipolar illness is usually best treated with an educational rather than a psychodynamic approach. This illness seems less dependent on external events and styles of interacting, and more on chemical imbalances. It is also a chronic and recurrent illness that will not disappear, and it requires ongoing treatment to help you cope. When you suffer from bipolar illness, at the beginning of an episode you may have little insight that you are ill. The mood distorts your perceptions so that you see the world as all-wonderful or all-terrible, and you cannot be reasoned out of this perception by conventional talking therapy. One of the signs that you are recovering from an episode is an awareness of how ill you have been.

A family-focused approach to education about the illness can be very helpful. Most families don't know much about bipolar disorder. Intense emotional interactions can make your condition worse. Once your family understands that your illness is caused by chemical imbalances, and not by flaws in the family, they can let go of their guilt and overinvolvement. Lowering the emotional temperature may give you space to calm down. If you have bipolar disorder you may be sensitive to overstimulation, and function better with low-key styles of emotional expression, and large doses of approval and attention from your relatives. Family members can be taught to speak warmly, to listen, and to let you know frankly but respectfully when your behaviour upsets them.

They may also be able to help you work against the disorder. When they know that you are currently unable to deal with too many outside events, they can assist you in decreasing your expectations. For example, you may have to settle for less stressful and less challenging work; you may have to forget about long journeys with time changes that upset your sleep patterns. Watching for signs of relapse can become the work of everyone in the family, so that new episodes are treated early. Accepting the illness and the need for long-term treatment often takes a long time, but it's well worth the effort.

Recently, cognitive behavioural therapy has been adapted for the treatment of people with bipolar illness.

6
Medications and Other Therapies

The brain is one of the most complex organs ever studied by scientists. In this three-pound (1.5-kg) mass, one hundred billion nerve cells network with each other, sending information back and forth between cells in the brain and to the rest of the body. Our thoughts, experiences, memories and feelings are all stored in these nerve cells.

A message goes from one nerve cell to the next by a combination of electrical and chemical impulses. One nerve cell can connect with up to a thousand other nerve cells, so the number of circuits of possible information-sharing is astronomical. Each time an impulse moves between two cells, an alteration occurs in both cells.

The brain is changing and developing not only in childhood but throughout life. Year after year, we get rid of cells we no longer need and add cells if they are needed. Every experience alters the brain in some fashion.

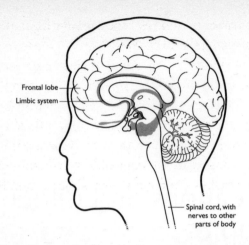

Frontal lobe

Limbic system

Spinal cord, with
nerves to other
parts of body

Mood disorders, such as depression and bipolar illness, are functional illnesses. When we call an illness functional, we mean that the changes are completely reversible. There is no permanent brain damage, as there would be from a stroke or a tumour. When the illness is treated, the brain again functions normally.

The regions of the brain important in understanding mood disorders are those involved in emotions, thoughts and memories. The limbic system, deep in the brain above the roof of the mouth, and its connection to the frontal lobe, the part of the brain behind the forehead, regulate our emotions and memories as well as basic functions like sleeping and eating. Other parts of the brain and body send messages to these two areas, either directly, through the nerve cells, or indirectly, through hormones in the bloodstream.

Picture the nerve cell as having many short 'legs', one very long 'leg', and a body in the middle. The short legs receive messages from other cells, and the one long leg delivers a message to the next cell. Messages travel in one direction only. The message passes through the legs by an electrical impulse which then passes out through the one long leg to the next cell. But there is a gap, called a synapse, between the two cells. When the electrical impulse reaches this gap, it changes to a chemical message, so it can cross the gap and reach the next cell. The receiving cell then translates the chemical message back into an electrical impulse, and the message travels through that cell too, and on and on. Of course, the messages travel through cells and across synapses at unimaginable speed; an impulse from your brain reaches your big toe in about a hundredth of a second.

The Brain in Depression

When the electrical message changes into a chemical message to cross the synapse, three small molecules, or neurotransmitters (NTs) – called norepinephrine, serotonin and dopamine – are involved. NTs are highly concentrated in two areas at the back of the limbic system. When there is a decrease in NTs at the synapse, we become depressed.

A group of drugs called antidepressants can help to decrease the intensity of depression when they are taken in pill, capsule or liquid form daily for four to eight weeks. They are thought to work at the synapse by increasing the concentration of NTs. But this alone does not stop depression. The next necessary step happens in the cell wall on the receiving side of the gap, which has receptors to receive the NTs' message. The receptors and the NTs fit into each other like the pieces of a jigsaw puzzle. Different receptors are involved in different actions; we label the various kinds with numbers such as 2 and 3. Since the depressed brain has too few NTs in the gap, the number of receptors on the wall of the receiving cell greatly increases, so

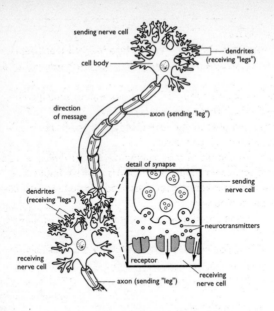

Nerve cells and synapse

these receptors can grab the scarce NTs going by. Once antidepressants increase the supply of NTs in the gap, the receiving cell can 'relax' and the number of receptors can decrease. At this point, the depression improves. This whole process takes four to eight weeks before the antidepressant really works.

This is the current theory of depression, and how antidepressants help. Keep in mind, though, that scientists are constantly making new discoveries, and adjusting the theory.

Antidepressants

In the late 1950s, the first antidepressant, imipramine, was identified. At almost the same time, iproniazide, a drug used to treat tuberculosis, was found to have antidepressant

---

Drug groups

These are generic names of some drugs used to treat depression. For brand names, please see the drug table near the end of the book.

- tricyclic antidepressants (TCAs): imipramine, amitriptyline, clomipramine, nortriptyline, desipramine
- monoamine oxidase inhibitors (MAOIs): phenelzine, tranylcypromine, iproniazide
- reversible inhibitors of monoamine oxidase (RIMAs): moclobemide
- selective serotonin reuptake inhibitors (SSRIs): fluoxetine, fluvoxamine, paroxetine (not prescribed for under 18-year-olds), sertraline, citalopram
- norepinephrine and dopamine reuptake inhibitors (NDRIs): bupropion
- serotonin-norepinephrine reuptake inhibitors (SNRIs): venlafaxine
- serotonin-2 antagonist/reuptake inhibitors (SARIs): trazodone
- serotonin 2,3 antagonist and serotonin-norepinephrine reuptake inhibitors (SA/SNRIs): mirtazapine

---

properties. After these two drugs were discovered, other antidepressants were developed that had fewer side effects, more sedation, quicker onset of action, and other preferable characteristics. Research continues to come up with faster-acting and better antidepressants. The drugs are used for depression, and are also used – combined with mood-stabilizing drugs – for the depression phase of bipolar disorder.

In treating depression, we want to increase the level of NTs in the synapse (gap). How can we do that? It's a complicated process, but if you have a basic understanding of how it works, the different groups of antidepressants will be much easier to understand.

In cells on the 'sending' side of the synapse, enzymes convert certain molecules into the NTs epinephrine and serotonin. These are released into the synapses to do their 'messenger' work. But they don't remain active indefinitely. They are deactivated in one of two ways: either they are taken back (*reuptake*) into the 'sending' cells and deactivated there, or an enzyme called *monoamine oxidase* (MAO) deactivates them within the synapse. They are eventually metabolized, or broken down, by the liver and kidneys. By slowing down the deactivation of NTs while new ones are being created, we can increase the level of NTs in the synapses at any given time.

We use various groups of drugs to slow down the decrease of NTs in specific ways. We can inhibit (block) the reuptake of NTs by the sending cells, by using drugs that fool the body. We can inhibit the breakdown action of the MAO. Or, if we want to stop the action of some receptors but not others – for example, if we want to block depression without causing nausea or sexual dysfunction – we can use an *antagonist* to target specific receptors. Thus, a drug described as a *serotonin-2 antagonist/reuptake inhibitor* stops the action of the number-2 receptors in the receiving cells, while also blocking the deactivation of the serotonin so that it remains active longer.

Interactions and Side Effects

Other drugs or foods competing for enzymes in the liver, or damage to the liver itself, can delay the metabolism of a drug so that the drug stays at a high level for a long time. Kidney damage can also raise the level of drug in the blood. Both the time of day the drug is taken and whether it is taken on a full or empty stomach can change the amount and rate of absorption as well. Drugs are metabolized at different rates in different people; a small dose may be as effective in some people as a large dose in others. This variation depends not only on obvious differences, such as weight and height, but also on age, race and sex. In the past, most dosages were calculated for the average-size white male. In 1993, legislation was introduced in the United States so that the drug trials run by pharmaceutical companies before the drug was marketed had to consider dosages for females as well. Blood tests during these trials measure the level of drug in the blood, allowing for further fine-tuning.

All the cells of the body use NTs to conduct information, not just those in the brain. Therefore, medications affecting the level of NTs may also affect the stomach, the muscles, the urinary tract, the sex organs, the eyes, and many other systems. Some of the side effects are minor and fairly predictable; even if they make you uncomfortable, you need not stop the drug. These side effects are not dangerous and they usually diminish in a week or so. But if you develop a more serious reaction, such as a skin rash, severe infection, jaundice, or a marked decrease in urination, you should stop the drug and call your doctor, or go to the A & E department of your local hospital, right away.

Do not stop these medications because you feel a bit better and think you don't need them anymore. If you stop them for even a few days, the changes in the cells will stop and you will have to start the process all over again. Since it can take four to eight weeks to get the medication's full effect, this will be very discouraging. Studies show that only about 60 per cent of people end up properly taking the drugs they are prescribed, for either medical or psychiatric illnesses.

For example, Dorothy was prescribed paroxetine for severe, debilitating depression. She took it for three weeks, but stopped taking the medication a week before her appointment with the therapist because she hadn't noticed any improvement. She was alarmed by darting electric shock–like feelings in her head. As soon as she restarted the paroxetine, these disappeared; they had been a withdrawal reaction to the abrupt stopping of paroxetine. Her doctor gradually reduced the dose over a three-week period, so she wouldn't have withdrawal effects. Since the paroxetine had not been effective for Dorothy, she started on another antidepressant, and her depression lifted over the next three weeks.

If the drugs are working, you will first notice an improvement in sleeping and eating, and then a sense of calm, so that you are less upset by stresses. After about four weeks you will notice your mood improve. At first, be cautious about activities that require alertness and coordination. If you like a glass of wine when you go out with friends, it's probably best to forgo it when you first start the medication. It's also probably safer not to drive until you are familiar with the effects of the drug. If you are very agitated or unable to sleep, your doctor may prescribe a mild tranquilizer or sleeping pill until the antidepressant takes effect.

Millie came to see her doctor complaining of a ten-pound (5-kg) weight loss, early-morning wakening, agitation, fatigue, difficulty concentrating, and guilty feelings about an abortion she had had twenty years previously that she couldn't stop thinking about. She felt that life was not worth living, but had no plans to kill herself. She had been depressed and listless for about a month. Her doctor diagnosed a major depression and chose to start her on venlafaxine at a dose of 75 mg daily.

Within four days, Millie called saying she was more agitated and didn't feel she could continue on the medication. She had also thrown up a couple of times. The doctor suggested that she continue the medication but take the dose on a full stomach after her supper. When she returned to the clinic for her next appointment, she said she was feeling a bit less frightened and was sleeping longer. Her appetite had returned and she had not lost any more weight. She was told to increase the dose to 150 mg daily. Three weeks later, she reported that she was beginning to feel more like her old self.

If you don't feel any better after about six to eight weeks, then another drug, usually from the same group, can be tried. If there is some change but not as much as you would like, the antidepressant effect can sometimes be increased by adding an augmenting drug such as lithium, tryptophan – an amino acid that metabolizes (is converted) into the NT serotonin – or the hormone thyroxin. Your doctor can also prescribe antidepressants from two different groups at the same time, or a 'dual-action' drug that fits into more than one group.

Note that you will not develop tolerance or addiction to antidepressants. You will gradually feel better, but not 'high'. If you do feel elated on antidepressants, you may be developing hypomania (bipolar II, or 'soft' bipolar disorder), or mania, and the addition of a mood stabilizer will help.

Groups of Antidepressants and How They Work

TRICYCLICS (TCAs)

The tricyclic group of antidepressants – named for the three rings making up the chemical shape of the drug – act by blocking the reuptake of norepinephrine back into the sending cell, so there are more NTs in the gap to combat depression. Commonly prescribed drugs from this group include imipramine, amitriptyline, clomipramine, and newer compounds that have a quicker onset of action and fewer side effects, such as nortriptyline and desipramine. The doctor may need to increase the dosage of the drug until you get the full benefit.

Tricyclics have many possible side effects. Some of the more unwelcome ones are weight gain, drowsiness, constipation, dry mouth, blurred vision, dizziness and a decrease in blood pressure. You must move very slowly from lying down to sitting up to standing, so that your blood pressure can adjust to the change in posture; otherwise, you may faint. If you suffer from glaucoma (elevated pressure within the eyes) or heart problems, you may not be able to take these drugs. An overdose of tricyclics can be deadly.

Tricyclics work particularly well in depressed adult men, in severe depressions with many physical symptoms, and in depressions marked by excessive fatigue and lethargy. They are less often used in the young and the elderly because they slow the conduction time of the heart, increase the heart rate, and cause a lowering of the blood pressure.

Overdoses of small amounts of tricyclic antidepressants can be lethal particularly when combined with other mood altering substances such as alcohol. They can also be very risky in patients with major mental disorders such as schizophrenia and mania because of the risk of suicide. In bipolar patients, manic episodes can be started after taking any antidepressant. (See Bipolar Treatment).

Newer antidepressants are safer in overdoses and just as effective.

MONOAMINE OXIDASE INHIBITORS (MAOIs)

Monoamine oxidase inhibitors work by irreversibly changing the enzyme, monoamine oxidase, that breaks down NTs, so that amounts of both norepinephrine and serotonin increase in the synapses. Drugs in this group include phenelzine and tranylcypromine. These drugs are now used less frequently than in the past because they can be quite dangerous. They cannot be used with other antidepressants.

They cause the 'cheese reaction', a hypertensive (high blood pressure) crisis, when combined with certain foods – ripe cheeses, beer, liqueurs, offal, smoked meats, smoked fish, soy sauce, teriyaki, tofu, sauerkraut, fava beans, avocados, dried figs, caviar, yeast extracts such as Marmite and Bovril. These foods contain large amounts of the amino acid tyramine.

MAOIs also interact with off-the-shelf nasal sprays, cough medicines, and weight-control preparations containing ephedrine, and with other antidepressants such as the tricyclics and the selective serotonin reuptake inhibitors. If monoamine oxidase is irreversibly changed, the amino acid tyramine makes more and more norepinephrine, and there is no longer monoamine oxidase to inactivate it – or to inactivate ephedrine, which is very similar in action to norepinephrine. Eventually the level of norepinephrine becomes high enough to raise the blood pressure to the point where it causes a splitting headache or even a stroke. This is obviously a medical emergency. (Needless to say, your doctor would have to be certain you were not suicidal when using such a high-risk drug.) Some doctors even suggest you carry an antidote, phento-lamine, in case you have a sudden rise in blood pressure from a cheese reaction. In any case, if you have the reaction, you should go to the nearest A & E department at once.

REVERSIBLE INHIBITORS OF MONOAMINE OXIDASE (RIMAS)
The only drug in this category at present is moclobemide. Like the MAOIs mentioned above, this drug stops the enzyme monoamine oxidase from acting, but in this case the action is reversible. The blood pressure stays normal, and the drug works well at high doses. It is relatively free of uncomfortable side effects, although it can cause a dry mouth, blurred vision

and headaches. It should not be combined with antidepressants from other groups.

Selective Serotonin Reuptake Inhibitors (SSRIs)

Advances in chemistry now allow drug manufacturers to develop compounds that help with depression but have fewer uncomfortable side effects. These are the first of the so-called designer drugs. The molecules of these drugs are shaped similarly to the molecules of the NT serotonin, and can fool the body by replacing serotonin in the receptors of the nerve cells. By doing so, these drugs can block the reuptake of serotonin. Fluoxetine, fluvoxamine, paroxetine, sertraline and citalopram belong to this group. SSRIs are the antidepressants of choice if you are agitated and irritable, because they have a calming effect. They seem to work best in adult premenopausal women who are depressed.

These medications may cause a number of side effects, such as headache, nausea, dry mouth, sedation, dizziness, tremor, night sweats and sexual difficulties. About 30 per cent of people cannot have orgasms when taking these medications, because the receptor that activates orgasms in both sexes is blocked or inactivated, although these people still feel sexual desire. SSRIs are deactivated in the liver by a group of enzymes, the P450 enzymes, that also deactivate many foods, toxins and other medications. These enzymes can be overloaded, so that the level of SSRIs in the blood increases.

SSRIs work within a fairly predictable range of dosage, so your doctor will not need to keep raising the dosage to find a level that works. Another big advantage of the SSRIs is their safety in overdoses; prescribing for the depressed, suicidal patient is less risky.

Since the SSRI's have been available for longer periods,

doctors and consumers are becoming more aware of potential problems with these medications. It is important not to throw the baby out with the bath water. When used appropriately and judiciously, these medications can be life-savers but they are not panaceas for any unhappiness.

Serotonin Syndrome

Excess stimulation of serotonin causes this serious syndrome characterized by euphoria, drowsiness, overactive reflexes, abnormal muscle contractions in the jaw and foot, sweating, confusion and high body temperature. Combinations of drugs, overdoses and compromised liver or circulation problems can cause this medical emergency. The drugs are withdrawn immediately. Treatment in hospital is necessary as the condition can cause death. It is very important to tell your doctor about any other drugs you are taking in addition to SSRIs.

Herbal Medication and Over-the-counter Medications

More and more people are using over-the-counter medications and herbal remedies for symptoms of depression and anxiety. These compounds are chemicals and can cause side effects as well. Let your doctor know what other compounds you are taking even if it doesn't seem important. Many of these compounds can cause dangerous and even fatal reactions when combined with prescription drugs.

Withdrawal Syndrome

When someone has used SSRIs to treat depression and feel they no longer need the drug, they must decrease the dose very gradually over weeks or months to avoid very unpleasant withdrawal symptoms characterized by 'lightning-bolts in the head' or 'electric head' along with dizziness, mood swings, upset stomach and wildly unpleasant dreams. This is similar to withdrawal from addictive substances. However, these drugs differ from addictive substances as people do not develop dependency, that is, needing larger and larger amounts to achieve the same effect or euphoria, leading to psychological dependency.

Seroxat (paroxetine) and Effexor (venlafaxine) have been named as the most likely drug to cause withdrawal reactions if withdrawn too quickly according to the World Health Organization adverse drug reaction reports.

Ongoing Controversy about Treatment with SSRIs

Ever since the SSRIs were introduced, there have been anecdotal reports of suicide and violence amongst some people who have taken these drugs. No systematic studies to date support these claims. However, some people do develop an unpleasant, agitated feeling called 'akathisia' that may lead to suicidal feelings. In those cases, the drug should be immediately discontinued. Obviously, a research study designed to decide this controversy would be unethical.

In June 2003, the UK Medicines and Healthcare Products Regulatory agency (MARA) announced that paroxetine (Seroxat) should no longer be prescribed to patients under 18 years of age. This decision was quickly adopted in Canada and the USA as well. The study leading to this decision showed that children on paroxetine rather than a placebo experienced crying, mood changes, suicidal thoughts and attempts 3.2% of the time and the placebo group 1.5% of the time. No deaths were reported.

SSRIs have been very helpful for many patients. It is important that people understand the possibility of withdrawal symptoms developing on stopping an SSRI. Equally it is important that patients who have already shown suicidal or violent tendencies are carefully monitored for any behavioural changes once they begin taking these drugs.

NOREPINEPHRINE AND DOPAMINE REUPTAKE INHIBITORS (NDRIs)

Only one drug has been developed in this group, bupropion. It works well in bipolar depression but is very effective in all types of depression. This is the only antidepressant so far that works on the neurotransmitter dopamine, as well as norepinephrine. It has also been marketed to help people stop smoking. Side effects may include a dry mouth, increased perspiration, tremor, nausea and headache. One early study showed that people with bulimia who took bupropion developed seizures at dosages above 300 mg. (Bulimia is an eating disorder in which a person induces vomiting after eating in order to control weight.) The usual dose is 150 to 300 mg daily.

SEROTONIN-NOREPINEPHRINE REUPTAKE INHIBITORS (SNRIs)

Again, only one drug, venlafaxine, fits this category. It tends to block the reuptake of serotonin at lower doses, and the reuptake of both norepinephrine and serotonin at higher doses, above 225 mg a day. The drug is very effective because of this dual action. Possible side effects include dry mouth, increased perspiration, sedation and sexual difficulties, similar to those encountered with the SSRIs. Hypertension can also be a problem at high doses and blood pressure needs to be monitored.

SEROTONIN-2 ANTAGONIST/REUPTAKE INHIBITORS (SARIs)
This group of drugs helps if you are prone to developing sexual difficulties from the SSRIs. One is available, trazodone. It is an effective antidepressant with many of the same properties as the SSRIs, such as safety and effectiveness, without the sexual difficulties, because it affects serotonin in a different way. It can cause nausea, dry mouth and sedation. However, it causes priapism in one case in eight thousand. (Priapism is a sustained erection that cannot be softened and can be very painful.)

SEROTONIN 2,3 ANTAGONIST AND SEROTONIN-NOREPINEPHRINE REUPTAKE INHIBITOR (SA/SNRI)
The one drug in this group, mirtazapine, is the newest antidepressant to be approved for use in the UK. It has the advantage of causing very little sexual dysfunction and nausea because it does not inactivate the receptors involved in these side effects. It causes an increase of the neurotransmitters norepinephrine and serotonin. It only has to be taken once a day, at bedtime. Since it causes sleepiness in 54 per cent of people, this can help those who have difficulty sleeping when they are depressed. Within two weeks of starting treatment, the sleep disturbances and anxiety of depression are lessened. Unfortunately, mirtazapine also causes weight gain in 12 per cent of users – but nothing's perfect.

Combining two antidepressants – one increasing the concentration of serotonin and one increasing the concentration of norepinephrine – is quite effective in treating depression until the person is free of symptoms.

The Brain in Bipolar Illness

If you have a bipolar illness, the depression looks the same as in depressive disorder but the treatment is different. The illness is not usually recognized and treated until about eight years after the first episode, and there may have been life-threatening suicide attempts by that time. Once the disorder is recognized, a mood stabilizer such as lithium is started. Lithium may act by opening channels in the receiving nerve cell, so that NTs can get through. It may also increase the number of brain cells in the limbic system, which tend to decrease after repeated depressions. At this point, both of these possibilities are theoretical only.

We do know that, when someone with bipolar disorder takes lithium as prescribed, episodes are six times less frequent and the risk of suicide is ten times lower. Unfortunately, lithium has a narrow therapeutic safety zone, meaning that the effective dose is only about half of the lethal dose. That's why, if you are taking lithium, it's important to have the level of lithium in your blood checked regularly. In the summer, when you lose salt (sodium chloride) through perspiring, it's important to replace the sodium with drinks like ginger ale and lemonade; lithium fills in for missing sodium and will build up to toxic levels when your sodium is low. Some of the side effects you should watch for if you are on lithium are fatigue or lethargy, clouded thinking and impaired concentration, severe nausea and vomiting, dizziness, muscle weakness, slurred speech and unsteady walk. If you start to have these symptoms, stop taking the medication and call your doctor or go the A & E department.

Lithium can affect other systems of the body, such as the thyroid gland, the kidneys and the heart. Before starting you on

Danger signs for lithium users

The following warning signs may indicate a toxic buildup of lithium. If you develop any of these, stop taking the lithium, and go to your doctor or a hospital A & E department immediately.

• fatigue or lethargy
• clouded thinking and impaired concentration
• severe nausea and vomiting
• dizziness
• muscle weakness
• slurred speech
• unsteady walk

the drug, your doctor will probably check these systems to make sure you can tolerate the medication. If you develop severe vomiting and diarrhoea due to a virus, if you go for long periods without drinking fluids, or if you exercise excessively, particularly in high temperatures, it is very important to replace the water and salt that your body has lost.

At first, you may not like taking lithium because you miss the 'highs' of the mood swings. In the long run, though, you may find the trade-off worthwhile. If you have a bipolar illness and you don't take mood stabilizers, you will probably spend much more time in an incapacitating depressed or mixed state than in an exhilarated manic or hypomanic state.

Some doctors think it is better to treat the depression of bipolar illness by adding the antidepressant bupropion to lithium, rather than adding another mood stabilizer. Valproic acid can cause liver damage at normal levels. Carbamazepine can cause a sudden shutdown of the production of blood cells by the bone marrow in one person in twenty thousand taking this drug.

Drugs to Control Symptoms

In addition to the drugs that treat depression directly, there are a number of medications that can help relieve symptoms.

Minor Tranquilizers and Sedatives

A minor tranquilizer can decrease anxiety for about four to six hours. A sedative acts longer and is strong enough to cause sleep. In depression, insomnia and anxiety can be upsetting problems. You may notice a change in your sleep pattern when another episode is beginning. Treating the sleep disturbance and anxiety with faster-acting drugs, before the anti-depressants take effect, can help. For the sleep disturbances, a mild tranquilizer at bedtime may be enough. For more severe depressions, a stronger medication such as a sedative at bedtime may be necessary.

Many tranquilizers and sedatives belong to the benzo-diazepine group of drugs, which alter your sleep patterns and can cause addiction. In addition, they act for short periods, so that when the effects wear off you can end up feeling lower than ever. Despite these drawbacks, the drugs can be useful for short periods.

A new type of sedative, called zopiclone, is safer to use because it does not interfere with sleep patterns. A new type of anxiety-relieving drug, called buspirone, does not cause addiction but must be taken regularly to be effective.

Major Tranquilizers

Your doctor may suggest major tranquilizers if you are having psychotic symptoms, such as mania or psychotic depression, or if you are experiencing severe agitation and sleeplessness that cannot be otherwise controlled. Two newer medications in this group, risperidone and olanzapine, have been shown to have less serious side effects than older choices such as chlorpromazine or haloperidol. After prolonged use, these older drugs can lead to a permanent neurological disorder called tardive dyskinesia, which causes involuntary twitching movements of the face that are permanent and disfiguring. There is no known treatment. Unfortunately, weight gain is a fairly common side effect of both risperidone and olanzapine. A newer drug, quetiapine, does not cause weight gain. Atypical antipsychotics are now being recommended as a useful addition in the treatment of bipolar mood disorders both in the depressive and manic phase.

Antidepressants not recommended

Most antidepressants can induce a manic or hypomanic episode if given to a patient with bipolar illness. If at all possible, the doctor will try to avoid using them.

Other Physical Treatments for Depression

There are a number of non-drug treatments that may help relieve depression.

Electroconvulsive Therapy (ECT)

In the 1930s, electroconvulsive therapy was noted to improve severe depression. The therapy was based on the mistaken notion that people with epilepsy did not get depressed, perhaps because of the repeated convulsions they experienced. At the time electroconvulsive therapy was first developed, few treatments were available for depressive illness.

Since antidepressants became available in 1959, ECT has been used less. However, it works well for some types of illness, and is particularly useful in certain conditions. If you are psychotically depressed with terrifying delusions and hallucinations, if you are determinedly suicidal, if you are severely debilitated from malnutrition, if you have heart disease, or if you are pregnant and can't take medications, it may be your best choice. The procedure is physically safe and works much more rapidly than antidepressants.

The person is given muscle relaxants and anaesthesia. Then an electrical impulse is administered to the skin of the skull to induce a seizure. The electrical impulse may be delivered to one side of the brain, the non-dominant hemisphere, to minimize memory loss. Treatments are usually given about twice a week over a three-week or five-week period. Symptoms start to improve by the second or third treatment.

Opposition to the use of electroconvulsive therapy has been heated during the last few decades. The procedure sounds alarming in an era when pills are expected to cure everything. Consumer groups saw ECT as an assaultive and hurtful procedure and worked to have it abolished as a form of treatment. The National Institute for Clinical Excellence produces regular advice on the modes of administration and an audit of effectiveness, both from hospitals and patient groups.

However, there is strong evidence that ECT is an effective and life-saving procedure when appropriately used.

Transcranial Magnetic Stimulation

This newer and less invasive method of electrostimulation was developed recently as an alternative to ECT. It's still in the investigative stage, but seems to have possibilities for treating depression safely. During positron emission tomography (PET), a type of diagnostic scan that shows the activity of the brain, it was noted that depressive patients had less blood flow to the frontal lobes of the brain than non-depressive people. When a low-level electrical current is applied to the left side of the head in the frontal area, once a day for two weeks, the blood flow to the area increases, and the depression improves.

Intravenous Hydrocortisone

When someone is exposed to repeated stresses, the body's steroid hormones, which are produced by the adrenal gland in response to stress, may become depleted. This depletion can lead to depression. Hydrocortisone, a form of steroid, can be injected to correct this situation, leading to a 50 per cent improvement in symptoms almost immediately.

Light Therapy

In 1898, the Antarctic explorer Dr Frederick Cook wrote that the winter darkness at the pole left 'people in a condition similar to that of a plant deprived of direct sunlight, that the presence of the sun is as essential to animal life as it is to vegetable life.'

Northern climates have weak sunlight during the day, as well as shorter days, in the winter months. Some people – more women, particularly during child-bearing years, than men – become depressed with this decrease in light. Their daily rhythm cycle is disrupted and they develop a variant of depression called seasonal affective disorder (SAD). SAD is often accompanied by eating disorders and/or premenstrual dysphoria syndrome (PMS).

Phototherapy (light therapy) helps counter the effects of decreased light. The person sits in front of a special lamp for 30 to 60 minutes at the same time each day – preferably in the morning – during the winter months. There's no need to stare into the light; it's fine to read the newspaper over a cup of tea. The lamp mimics daylight by emitting 2,500 to 10,000 lux, and adjusts the activity of the brain's sleep-wake cycle. These lights can be purchased in the UK. You can ask your doctor for the name of a local distributor. (A winter trip to the Caribbean would work wonders as well. Too bad your health plan won't cover it!)

7
Complementary Treatments and Self-Help

Phillipa was a sixty-eight-year-old widow who had lost her husband after a lengthy illness three years previously. She was lonely, fearful and desolate. She and her husband had been active politically, they had had lively dinner parties and discussion groups with colleagues, but all that had ceased with his death. She was convinced that she was a burden to her children and friends, so she stayed home by herself. She didn't feel well, and had to rest often during the day. She had been to several doctors but they didn't really seem to listen to her complaints, and no explanation was found for her fatigue and weakness. Eventually Phillipa was placed on low doses of an antidepressant that improved her mood somewhat. She got up the energy to visit a massage therapist and an acupuncturist. Both these practitioners seemed much more responsive and interested in her concerns than the doctors had been and, with regular visits, she began to feel better.

Complementary Treatments

There are a number of supportive therapies that may be helpful when you are depressed. Alternative methods can offer many advantages. Most are directed at the whole person, integrating body, mind and spirit, and take advantage of the innate healing ability of the body. Some are derived from Eastern religions and spiritual sources. Others are folkloric remedies that have been handed down from ancient times.

In 1990, 34 per cent of people in the United States and Canada used alternate healing. By 1997, the proportion had increased to 50 per cent. In 2001, a UK postal survey found that 42 per cent of respondents had used alternative therapies for mental health problems. The reasons most frequently cited for visiting an alternative healer are fatigue, headaches, insomnia, depression and anxiety.

Dr Candice Pert, a neuroscientist who discovered the opiate receptor in the brain when she was doing research at the US National Institute of Mental Health, has developed a theory that integrates alternative and traditional healing methods and strives to account for the body's own healing ability. She thinks endokines, chemicals that travel throughout the bloodstream, carry messages about the emotional state of the body to all the cells affected in the body and brain. She believes that messages about the emotions are sent back and forth so adjustments can be made between the various parts of the system. Neurotransmitters and hormones are both types of endokines. When the delicate balance of endokines is upset by the introduction of external chemicals, such as alcohol and cocaine, emotions may be dramatically altered, and it may take a great deal of time and effort to restore that balance. Methods used by natural healers – such as massage, acupuncture, therapeutic touch, meditation, guided imagery and relaxation – probably help to right the balance of the endokine system. Many of these methods are rhythmic, repetitive and sensuous, soothing the person much as good mothering does.

Physical Therapies

Endorphins are naturally occurring opioids that the brain produces. They make us feel better, and they may help in depression by improving our mood, at least temporarily. Exercise is thought to release endorphins, and vigorous aerobic exercise three or four times a week has been shown to counter mild to moderate depression. When we are depressed, however, we are likely to be totally incapable of performing vigorous aerobic exercise even once a week. For some of us it's not easy even when we aren't depressed.

Acupuncture and relaxation techniques probably help to improve mild depression, but studies have given inconsistent results. Although several studies compared acupuncture to the antidepressant imipramine, it is difficult to rule out the placebo effect with acupuncture – there's no practical way to compare people who have had acupuncture needles inserted to people who only *believe* they have! – and most of the studies have not been reproduced.

Meditation, massage therapy, aromatherapy and yoga can all be used to improve mood. They are not only for depression, but increase good feelings in healthy people as well. A study on adolescents showed that music and massage therapy improved the brainwave patterns associated with depression. Any of these approaches may be helpful, and none is likely to do harm, but be sure to consult your doctor before trying them.

Herbs and Supplements

Over the years, many folkloric and herbal remedies have entered the list of drugs used by mainstream medicine. Aspirin was taken from the bark of the white willow tree; North American aboriginals made a tea out of this bark to treat fevers. Digoxin, a medicine used to treat heart failure, was developed from the foxglove plant. Vincristine, an anticancer drug, came from the periwinkle.

One of the herbal compounds used most frequently for depression is St John's wort, which is available off the shelf at chemists and health-food shops. This plant was known in Greek times; Hippocrates thought it was helpful in treating depression. The active ingredient, hypericum, has been shown to improve depression in some studies, but the evidence is not consistent. A 1996 analysis of twenty-three studies suggested that St John's wort was effective in treating depression. A recent, more carefully controlled study in American universities concluded that there was no significant effect. This product is currently the best-selling antidepressant in Germany. The recommended dosage to improve depression is 100 to 300 mg daily, divided into three doses, of a 3 per cent concentration of hypericum. Sedation and photosensitivity (an increased chance of sunburn) are two possible side effects at this dose. St John's wort can interact with other herbal remedies, such as chamomile, valerian and ginseng, to cause sedation, altered states of consciousness and decreased alertness. As well, the effect of prescription antidepressants is exaggerated in someone who is already taking St John's wort.

Valerian root, used since Greek and Roman times to induce sleep and decrease anxiety, is also available off the shelf. However, people who are sensitive to this compound can suffer liver damage even at average doses. If excessive amounts are used, anyone can develop headaches and excitability.

Melatonin is an amino acid that is sold in health-food stores in the United States. It is produced internally in the body, by the pineal gland, to set the body's circadian (daily) rhythms. It has been recommended for people who suffer from jet lag, and it may also help with seasonal affective disorder. It is not currently available in the UK.

SAMe is a form of the amino acid methionine that has been sold in Europe by prescription to treat depression. Several studies have shown it to be effective in treating mild to moderate depression, but in very high doses; the dosage required costs about $30 US a day. Studies of SAMe's effectiveness are inconsistent, and some are too short in duration to be convincing. The amount of active ingredient varies greatly from brand to brand, and SAMe can interact adversely with other medications.

Eating specific foods may in certain cases help counter depression. Some depressed people are deficient in specific nutrients, even though they have no clinical signs such as anaemia. Two of the worst culprits are folic acid and vitamin B12. Other B vitamins, such as thiamine and niacin, are also thought to help counter depression. Some people are deficient in trace minerals such as zinc and magnesium. Essential amino acids and omega-3 fatty acids, found in fish oils, are also thought to help counter depression. If your diet

Be cautious with complementary therapies

Although many non-medical therapies can be helpful, there are some problems with these 'alternative' or complementary approaches. Some have not been thoroughly researched, so claims for their success rest on dubious theories or unreliable testimonials. Others are dangerous for people with certain medical conditions.

Some people think herbal products must be safe because they are natural compounds. The fact is, they do have side effects, and they do sometimes interact with each other or with prescription drugs; the combined effect may be unsafe. Also, because herbals don't yet have to meet health and safety standards (as prescription drugs do), the concentration of active ingredients may vary from none to far more than the package says – and the product may even be contaminated.

Consult your doctor about any complementary products and therapies you are considering, and choose them with caution and common sense.

includes whole, fresh foods from the fat, protein and carbohydrate food groups, you are probably getting adequate supplies of most of these elements, and it's unlikely that you require supplements. But it's very hard to prove or disprove the alleged effects of trace elements such as magnesium, zinc, manganese and bismuth, as we can't experiment by removing these elements from our diet to find out whether we will develop depression without them. Even if adding extra amounts makes us feel better, there may be other reasons – including the placebo effect – for the improvement. Cause and effect can't be proven.

All in all – if your doctor believes that a complementary therapy isn't hurting you, and if you feel better with it, that's fine. But if your doctor warns you against it – or if you are promised an instant cure for an excessive amount of money – beware. There are no 'magic bullets' for depression so far,

---

The placebo effect

Any treatment causes an improvement in about one third of patients, even if the treatment is no more than water or sugar pills, as long as the patient doesn't know that the treatment has no active ingredients. We call this the placebo effect, and we're not sure why it happens. Drug trials have to allow for the fact that some of the improvement observed will be due to the placebo effect. This effect also makes it harder to tell whether complementary therapies are really effective.

---

and the condition can make you very desperate. Don't make yourself more of a victim.

Self-Help

While you are waiting for the illness to go away, there are certain things you can do to make yourself feel better. You won't feel like following all these suggestions right away, but start with a few of the more palatable ideas and build up gradually. It's probably better to focus on doing some activities, even if they seem mundane. Brooding and ruminating about how awful you feel, and wondering why this is happening to you, doesn't help at all. Take a small step at a time, and don't expect to get better suddenly. You will gradually improve each day. Recovery from a major depressive episode takes a while.

Try not to make major decisions about your life until after the depression lifts. The job that seems unbearable or the partner who seems insensitive may not look so bad when you are less miserable. If things still look grim when you are feeling better, you can change your situation then.

Let yourself make use of help that is offered; spend time with family and friends, and talk about your feelings. People like to help, and it's all right to let them know you need them. Try to take some initiative each day, but be realistic about what you can manage. Sometimes it helps to break tasks up into small bits. That way you won't feel so overwhelmed. For example, Jane had been unable to go to work for several days because she just couldn't drag herself out of bed in the morning. It sometimes took until one or two in the afternoon before she could get showered and dressed. She didn't feel hungry and couldn't bear the thought of making a meal for herself. But Jane had experienced a major depression before, so she realized what was happening. She asked her friend Maria, who worked with her, to come over with some food, talk to the people at work, and arrange to take her for a doctor's appointment later that week. Maria was glad to help; her own sister had been severely depressed, so she knew how incapacitated Jane felt.

While you gradually get your life back together, you can do activities that make you feel better. Try to be nice to yourself. Take a short walk, draw a picture, relax in a hot bath, bake biscuits and eat them, watch a funny film, book a massage, buy some flowers and scented candles, breathe deeply, meditate, play your favourite music, exercise, play with your pet, or just rest and drink herbal tea. Nutritional meal supplements, available in tins or bars at your grocery or chemists, can tide you over until you are ready to cook balanced meals again. Ask your doctor or chemist to recommend some brands.

A Note to Family Members

Patience comes first. Try to remember that depression takes time to improve. Do your best to offer emotional support by listening carefully, validating feelings, encouraging activities, and giving lots of affection. Try not to preach; it won't help. You have to care when your loved one doesn't. Monitor medications, encourage treatment, and don't ignore suicide threats. It's a tough job, but take heart – the depressive episode *will* end.

Beware, though. Depressed people are notorious for rejecting the help they need. Realize that your loved one or friend would 'snap out of it' if he or she could, so don't waste time with platitudes. Listen to the feelings expressed, even if they make you uncomfortable. Just listening can be wonderfully helpful.

8

Depression in Children and Adolescents

Jasmine was seventeen and in her third year of secondary school when her favourite aunt died suddenly. Her parents both worked, and she was often alone in the evenings, so she had been in the habit of visiting her aunt on her way home from school each day. They would have long talks about work and life and friends. In fact, her aunt was her best friend.

Jasmine was tall for her age, and very pretty. In year 8 a girl in her class who was much shorter and not as pretty had begun to make fun of her. She and her friends had teased Jasmine cruelly in the halls and after school, to the point where she had been reluctant to go to school. In year 10 she had finally told her school guidance counsellor. The girl and her friends had been warned to stay away from her but, as a result, many of her classmates had avoided her as well.

Jasmine told her family doctor that she was sleeping

poorly and that her school marks had dropped. She was desperately lonely since her aunt's death. She felt helpless to change things in her life, and felt life was no longer worth living. Jasmine's doctor placed her on an anti-depressant. Slowly she began to sleep better and became less tearful. She shared her feelings and ideas with her doctor, and gradually began to feel she could try to meet new friends.

All of us hope our children will be healthy and happy. We feel wonderful when they are secure and sociable, enjoying friends and activities and being curious to learn. Unfortunately, we aren't always able to protect them from upsetting experiences and feelings. Sometimes, all we can do is deal with the setbacks when they happen.

Depression in children seems to be on the increase. Between the ages of nine and seventeen at least 21 per cent of children show some emotional problems, and about 11 per cent have significantly impaired functioning at home, at school, and with their friends. The good news is that the disorder responds to treatment.

Sometimes depression in children appears similar to the adult illness, but more often your child's level of development determines how it looks. You may have trouble deciding whether your child needs treatment or is just going through a developmental stage that will pass. If your three-year-old has a temper tantrum, you expect it. If your eight-year-old behaves the same way, you start to worry.

Ahmed was three-and-a-half when his mother was killed in a car accident. His parents had divorced and his father had remarried and lived at the other end of the country. He and his new wife took custody of Ahmed, although previously they had seen him for only brief periods. At first Ahmed seemed contented enough, but within a week or two he started to have nightmares and would call out in his sleep. He would sob for long periods during the night, but would arch his back and pull away if his father or stepmother tried to comfort him. He seemed inconsolable. Both parents were aware that the loss of his mother was overwhelming for him, but eventually they became exhausted by his whining and demanding behaviour. Nothing seemed to make him happy. He began wetting his pants, and sometimes even messing his pants, although he had been completely toilet trained. His stepmother had not had children, and was looking forward to having her own. His father felt they had to put any plans to have children on hold because Ahmed's needs were paramount. This tension between the parents only made matters worse.

Ahmed was finally assessed at the local child guidance clinic. The parents were interviewed with him, to discuss their frustrations and sense of helplessness. Up to this time, no one had talked to Ahmed about his mother, for fear of upsetting him further. The animosity between Ahmed's natural parents had made it hard for his father to be neutral when discussing his ex-wife, while she had kept the boy from visiting his father and getting to know him. Finally, with the counsellor's help, the couple was able to accept Ahmed's need to grieve for his mother, and to make him feel welcome and safe in his new home. The symptoms decreased, but it was a long time before they disappeared.

Possible Signs of Childhood Depression

Your child may be whiny and clinging, or irritable and peevish. You may hear complaints of stomachaches and headaches. The child will sometimes describe unhappy feelings if asked directly. He or she may refuse to play with old friends, and may no longer seem to have any fun. Two-thirds of the time, the child will be struggling with other problems as well as depression. There may be a learning problem, incapacitating anxiety, eating problems, drug problems, trouble getting along with other children, or an attention deficit disorder that makes it difficult for the child to control his or her behaviour. According to an Ontario study, over 70 per cent of children with depression and other mental disorders do not get the help they need, either because the illness isn't recognized or because help isn't available.

If serious symptoms such as weight loss or suicidal thoughts or actions are present, you can easily tell your child needs help. In less clear cases, you have to decide how persistently unhappy your child is, and how much difficulty he or she has enjoying friends, managing in school, and getting along at home.

Causes of Depression in Children and Adolescents

How could your child develop such an illness? Many different factors, acting together, cause depression. The child's complicated makeup, including genetic endowment, physical health and psychological style, all contribute. The child's environment also plays a role. He or she interacts with – and over time is shaped by – you, siblings, friends, school and the community. The age and the timing of difficulties in the child's life, and the caretaking environment provided at home, can help or hinder the child's resilience.

Heredity plays a major role in the development of depressive disorders and bipolar disorders in children and adolescents. Of children with depression, 20 to 50 per cent have a family history of depression. The frequency is even higher for children with bipolar illness.

If one parent suffers from depression, your child is three times more likely to have a mood disorder than children whose parents are not depressed. If the parent's depression started before thirty years of age, the chances are even higher. Parental depression can affect your child in other ways. The parent may be too tired to set limits, or may feel miserable and, as a result, be too strict when the child misbehaves on one occasion, and then guilty and too lenient the next time. This inconsistency can confuse the child.

A child's temperament is consistent throughout development. Some children have traits that work in their favour to fend off depression, such as even sleep rhythms, an easygoing disposition, curiosity and persistence. Some are adaptable, and have the ability to organize their world and 'right' themselves when problems develop. But others have difficulty adapting to changes, so that each new stage of life is stressful and upsetting. With too many changes and too little support, they may develop depression or other psychiatric problems.

Family difficulties can contribute to the onset of depression. Lack of give-and-take between you and your child can cause trouble, and so can a parent-child relationship complicated by neglect and violence. Witnessing spousal violence and very angry verbal disputes within the family can also lead to depression in a child. Loss of a parent's love through death, chronic illness or divorce can be very painful. Less serious but still difficult losses result from the death of a pet, the loss of a friend, a family move or the birth of a new sibling.

Disasters, both manufactured and natural – can shake the child's faith in the world and in his or her own security. Ongoing threats of war and terrorism may create an atmosphere of fear and doubt that is fertile ground for depression. Children are exposed to violence from television shows, including the news, and this violence can cause a warped view of the world.

Bullying at school can also make the child's life a nightmare and lead to depression. Often a child will suffer silently rather than let parents or teachers know how severe the bullying is, for fear of reprisals. Some young suicides have been victims of persistent bullying.

Some child psychiatrists feel that the incidence of depression in children may be increasing because they have fewer supports than in the past. Many parents have less time to spend with their children, and are reluctant to set limits and clear expectations of behaviour when they are home because they want what time they have together to be easy and fun.

Children who have a delay in language development, both in speaking clearly and in understanding or finding words, may have trouble making their needs known during the preschool years; the frustration may lead to tantrums and hitting. During school years, they may have difficulty learning, and may feel humiliated by not doing as well as their friends. If the problem is not recognized and dealt with, depression may develop as a result of their frustrations.

Children who are socially awkward find it hard to make friends. They may not be able to read nonverbal cues, so they can't anticipate what other people are feeling and respond appropriately. (Reading social cues is an inborn skill, like language development.) Their social failure can lead to lowered self-esteem and possibly depression, if it is not dealt with. These children may be withdrawn, may not listen or cooperate with other children when playing, and may end up getting into trouble with schoolteachers and parents because of their uncooperative and unsociable behaviour.

Some children have a pessimistic thinking style that can lead to depression; they always see the glass as half empty and expect the worst to happen. They feel personally responsible for disasters and helpless to influence what happens. They tend to use expressions such as 'Nothing I do is going to help', or 'Everything I do is wrong'.

Ten-year-old Paul and his mother came to a child guidance clinic because the school was concerned about his disruptive behaviour. He was defiant and had sworn at his teacher when she told him he had to stay in at recess. He had then left the school without permission. Instead of returning home, he had gone to a vacant construction site, and police officers in a passing patrol car had spotted him running along the high scaffolding; he would have had a dangerous fall if he had lost his balance.

Paul's mother said that, up until a few months ago, Paul had been a funny, warm little boy who loved to cuddle. But then her father, who had lung cancer, had moved into their home so she could nurse him. Paul's grandfather had died three months ago. Paul's father wouldn't come to the clinic because he said Paul was just a 'bad seed'. He was living at home but had met another woman and was unsure he wanted to continue with the marriage. He and Paul spent little time together. Paul was angry about his father's neglect, and would talk openly about not having any use for him.

Paul was tested to see if he was having academic problems. He tested in the superior range of ability to learn and had no signs of a learning disability. When he talked to the counsellor, he said he missed his grandfather because the latter had paid attention to him and had told good jokes. Paul said he didn't like the other children at his school because they were 'sissies'. He fought with his sister and complained that she was treated better than him. He seldom smiled or made eye contact and was not very talkative. He seemed tense and angry most of the time. He was restless and unfocused, even when playing.

Paul's dangerous behaviour escalated, despite the counselling sessions. One week he reported that his father had beaten him, and the child and family team of the local social services was called, but the parents denied that the father had touched him. Paul was placed in a specialized treatment unit for six months, during which time his father was required to attend sessions. Paul also attended social skills groups during this time. When he did well he was praised, and when he misbehaved he was punished consistently. After a while, Paul and his father started to do things together, and both parents attended sessions to learn to deal with Paul differently.

Paul's problem was hard to identify at first because he had depression overshadowed by a conduct disorder. The treatment he received in counselling and in the child and family consultation centre was appropriate for both disorders. His behaviour improved but he and his parents would have to remain in treatment to be sure Paul didn't get into more serious trouble as he entered his teenage years.

Depression at Different Ages

Depression looks different at different ages, because developmental stages affect the picture. If you think your child is depressed, or if a teacher has mentioned the possibility to you, you can ask for a thorough physical and psychological assessment to be done by a child psychiatrist. Your family doctor can arrange this for you.

Infants

Depression in infants is rare, and is usually a sign of serious problems. The infant will be listless and apathetic, feed poorly and be unresponsive to people. He or she may sleep poorly and cry and whine. The facial expression is apprehensive or expressionless. This condition is usually seen in overcrowded orphanages where there is little touching or holding of the infants. The condition is reversible; a child placed with a sensitive, stable, caring family can develop mentally and emotionally with no lasting problems. This is important to know if you are thinking of adopting from a developing country.

Preschoolers

Preschoolers have no concept of the future or of cause and effect, so they are unable to express complex feelings such as guilt. Instead, the distressed feelings are shown through behaviours and body discomforts. A preschooler who is depressed may be restless and overactive, and unable to enjoy playing any more. He or she will complain of aches and pains, particularly headaches and stomachaches, and may be whiny and clingy with you, and fearful of new situations. The child may also be irritable and have temper tantrums over minor frustrations. You may have trouble keeping your patience if nothing seems to make your child happy.

Children of Elementary-School Age

When school-aged children are depressed, they may be moody, irritable and very sensitive to any criticism or rejection. They drag themselves around, sleep poorly, have trouble getting up in the morning, and show little interest in friends or activities. If you ask them, they'll say they're unhappy. Their schoolwork may drop off suddenly, or they may refuse to go to school altogether. They may complain of physical symptoms such as headaches and stomachaches. They may get into trouble at home and at school because of provocative and aggressive behaviour, and may be irritable with other children as well. They may even run away from home, or make suicidal statements such as 'I wish I had never been born' or 'I hope I get run over by a car'. A more ominous sign of suicidal intent occurs when the child starts giving away favourite belongings.

Adolescents

At this age, the depressive picture can be very dramatic. Depressed adolescents may stay away from friends or join a deviant peer group. They may be irritable and moody, sleep for long periods, and have difficulty getting up in the morning. They are often bored and may neglect their appearance. Girls who are depressed often develop eating problems such as obesity, anorexia or bulimia. Both sexes feel very negative about themselves when they are depressed, do poorly in school, and often start using street drugs and alcohol to feel better temporarily. They can describe feeling unhappy, but they are often uncommunicative with their parents, teachers and other adults.

Girls tend to develop depression more often than boys. They seem more vulnerable to losses of relationships, and are more concerned about social competence. Also, girls tend to focus on hurtful events and ruminate about the outcomes.

Signs of an eating disorder

Anorexia and bulimia are most common in adolescent girls, but they can occur in either sex, in any age group. In anorexia the child's weight is far below normal as a result of intentionally eating very small amounts. In bulimia the child maintains a 'fashionable' weight by alternately binge eating and vomiting or purging. The child hides these behaviours from the parents, and can be quite ill by the time the disorder is discovered.

Some signs to watch for are:

- preoccupation with food and weight
- 'feeling fat' when weight is normal or low
- guilt and shame about eating
- excessive exercising
- absence of menstrual periods
- hair loss; yellow, pasty skin; fine hair over the whole body; bloating
- weight fluctuations; dental problems; swelling of salivary glands in the lower cheeks, giving a 'chipmunk' look; frequent vomiting after meals
- a perfectionist, rigid, self-critical attitude, especially about physical appearance
- strange rituals around eating, such as eating only certain foods, counting the bites, hiding food
- hiding thinness with bulky clothes

Their self-blame and helplessness can lead to depression. Hormonal changes after puberty further predispose girls to depression.

Bipolar Disorders

About 35 per cent of bipolar disorders begin in late adolescence, and there is evidence that some children develop the illness even before puberty. Anxiety disorders, attention deficit disorder, and substance abuse frequently indicate the presence of a bipolar disorder. When a child or teen develops this disorder, there is often a strong family history of bipolar disorder, suicide, or alcoholism.

Bipolar illness in adolescence is a serious disorder. About 63 per cent of those affected have delusions – fixed ideas that have no basis in reality – and about 50 per cent have hallucinations; that is, they hear voices or have visions that aren't there. Such an adolescent may show elation, euphoria and a heightened sense of well-being that can quickly be replaced by anger and irritability. Rapid speech with wordplay and puns is common, as are rhyming patterns and contrived sentences such as 'The big bad bod banged the bangle on the bingle.' The teen may rarely sleep, and may use street drugs to calm down; sometimes it's difficult to distinguish the effects of the street drugs from the symptoms of the illness. Any teenager who is confused and seems out of touch with reality should be taken to a hospital A & E department as soon as possible, because there may be a risk of suicide. It is a mistake to dismiss the symptoms as adolescent turmoil.

Treatment of Depression and Bipolar Disorder in Children and Adolescents

Severe, untreated depression can be life-threatening to a child. One in ten children who suffer a major depressive episode before puberty goes on to commit suicide as an adult. Adolescents who have one major depressive episode are three to four times more likely to have another major depressive episode. Adolescents who are depressed are three to four times more likely than their peers to abuse alcohol and drugs. The risk of completed suicide is also high. Early recognition and thorough treatment of this major public health problem can save lives and avoid a great deal of misery.

For mild depression, a counsellor can begin by meeting with the family and child regularly, to talk about the illness

---

Signs of substance abuse

A 1996 study in the United States found that, by the eighth grade, 26 per cent of adolescents had used alcohol and 11 per cent had used marijuana within the last thirty days. By twelfth grade, the use of alcohol had risen to 50 per cent and the use of marijuana to 21 per cent. The UK 2000 census found that 22.8% of adolescents had used marijuana over the previous year.

Some signs that your child may be using drugs are:
- a drop in school marks, poor attendance
- a change in friends
- uncharacteristic irritable behaviour, memory problems
- altered sleeping patterns, especially excessive tiredness
- stealing money
- suddenly having excessive amounts of money
- staying out without permission
- not telling you where he or she is
- withdrawal from family and regular friends
- altered awareness, disorientation

and teach the family about depression. Knowing what you are coping with can decrease the guilt and anger you are feeling, so you can start to deal with the illness without blame. A counsellor can also look for stresses that are affecting the child and making the depression worse; for example, the child's teacher may be asked to decrease homework assignments for a time. Another question is how difficulties in communicating and solving family problems may be affecting the child. If the child has other psychiatric problems, such as anxiety, a learning disability or attention deficit disorder, these conditions can be treated as well.

Other forms of therapy will help if the child is more depressed. Cognitive behavioural therapy has shown good results in children, particularly when conducted in groups. The children learn to question their pessimistic and self-deprecating thoughts, and they may have homework assignments to help them sort out why they see the world so negatively. The group interaction is helpful as teenagers are very good at picking up inconsistencies and false assumptions, and pointing them out to each other.

Social skills training is a method of teaching children how to interact with others in a constructive manner, how to control their impulsiveness and anger, and how to ask appropriately for what they need. Social skills groups teach children how to behave with other children so they will be included and liked. They also help children deal with frustration. The children learn to talk about feelings, rather than physically attack someone, when they are upset.

Interpersonal therapy has been modified for children and teenagers, and a protocol to meet the needs of a single-parent family has been developed. After all, three of the premises of interpersonal therapy – grief, role transitions and role disputes – are involved in separation and divorce. An open discussion and acknowledgment of the stresses can be very helpful to a child. When people are going through the turmoil and sadness of a divorce, they may have few resources left to help their children. Often the children are reluctant to admit how hurt they have been by the divorce, because they are aware of their parents' pain and they don't want to cause them further trouble.

Family therapy can also be helpful with children and teens. Often, discord in the family can best be dealt with by having each member of the family explain his or her point of view, and then sorting out the conflicts. The therapist acts as a mediator in the process, so that each member has a chance to be heard and understood.

For moderate and severe forms of depression that do not improve with therapy, antidepressant medication sometimes helps. Tricyclics such as imipramine and nortriptyline have

---

Signs of suicide risk in a child or teen
- dramatic change in personality
- conflict with, and withdrawal from, friends and family
- decreasing quality of schoolwork
- acting bored or having trouble concentrating
- acting rebellious in odd or extreme ways
- running away from home
- abusing drugs or alcohol
- complaining of headaches or stomachaches
- changing sleeping and eating habits
- worsening of physical appearance
- giving away favourite possessions
- writing notes or poems about death
- talking about suicide; saying 'I can't take it any more', 'No one cares about me'.
- previous suicide attempt

not been shown to work for the treatment of depression in children, and should probably not be prescribed, as they can interfere with the electrical signals that control the heartbeat. Fluoxetine has been shown to be moderately effective in depression in children. The SSRIs work well in adolescents, and are probably the drugs of choice for them. For a bipolar adolescent, the drug treatment is the same as for the bipolar adult discussed in Chapter 6. Paroxetine is not recommended for children under 18 years.

For severe depression – especially when there are serious thoughts of suicide, psychotic symptoms or a refusal to eat or drink – hospitalization may be necessary, to protect the child or adolescent.

Suicide in Children and Adolescents

If your child threatens suicide, take the threat seriously but calmly. For every hundred juvenile suicide attempts, there is one completed suicide. However, the suicide rate increased 300 per cent in the fifteen-to-nineteen age group between 1950 and 1990, and suicide is now the second-highest cause of death in this group, in the UK. Males complete suicide more frequently than females, but females attempt suicide more often. Overdosing on medication is the commonest method, and firearms are the most deadly.

Risk factors include a history of depression, a previous suicide attempt, a family history of depression and suicide, family disruption, physical illness, living in a group home, and previous physical and/or sexual abuse.

Teenagers who are concerned about their sexual orientation are three times more likely to commit suicide, but a child who is uncertain about sexual orientation rarely voices these concerns openly, for fear of disappointing his or her parents. If your teenager talks about friends who are struggling with sexual identity problems, it may be a clue. It's important to talk about sexual identity issues comfortably in the family, avoiding 'gay jokes' and disparaging remarks about homosexuals.

Conflicts with parents, a breakup of a relationship, or trouble in school or with the law can all precipitate a suicide attempt. In 50 per cent of these attempts, alcohol is involved. The adolescent may be trying to escape an intolerable living situation, to make someone see how desperate he or she feels, or to make someone feel sorry or guilty. Like depression in general, suicidal behaviour can be hereditary. Identical twins are three times as likely as fraternal twins to both try suicide. 'Cluster suicides' – a number of suicides in a school or community over a brief period of time – can occur.

If you suspect that your teenager is at risk, you can have him or her evaluated by a family doctor, or a clinic, or in an A & E department. These *threats must be taken seriously*. The person who examines your teen should ask directly if he or she has considered suicide, and has made definite plans. *Asking does not cause suicide*; instead, it gives the teen permission to talk about any 'insoluble problems'. When there is a serious risk of suicide, the doctor will tell your teenager that the information cannot be kept from you; the usual confidentiality of the physician-patient relationship no longer applies. If the doctor does not feel your teenager is safe to manage alone, the teen can be hospitalized until an assessment and management plan is put in place. This can even be done without your teenager's consent, for a short period, if the risk is serious enough.

9
Women and Depression

Women are twice as likely as men to suffer from major depression. Between the onset of menstruation and menopause, monthly cycles keep changing the levels of the female hormones, estrogen and progesterone, which can affect how women feel. During the last few decades, there have been rapid social changes in women's lives as well. Both the hormonal cycles and these social factors, acting together, give women a greater chance of becoming depressed.

Much has been written about the social changes in the lives of women in the last generation. Many women feel they have to measure up in a host of areas. To be a good mother, wife and daughter; a success at work; and attractive and slim, all at the same time, can be a bit much. Paradoxically, if your sense of worth comes from several roles at once, you are less likely to become depressed; setbacks in one area are often compensated for by success in another. Mothers who work are depressed less often than those who stay at home, probably because, when they are having difficulties in one role, they still get a sense of satisfaction from another in which they think they are doing well.

Depression looks a little different in women than in men. It usually begins in late adolescence. Irritability and anxiety are prominent symptoms, rather than sadness and guilt. Diffuse aches and pains, fatigue, and sleeping and eating disturbances may all be present. Stress and feelings of helplessness seem to aggravate the symptoms.

Hormones

Let's follow the monthly hormone cycle starting when the period begins. The estrogen level starts low, increases through the next few days, and gradually peaks just before the egg is released from its sac in the ovary, halfway through the month. The pituitary gland, in the brain, secretes *follicle-stimulating hormone* so that the ovary will develop a mature egg that can be released into the uterus for fertilization. The empty follicle in the ovary is stimulated by *luteinizing hormone* from the pituitary gland to produce progesterone, which thickens the lining of the uterus so the egg can implant itself if it's fertilized. After ovulation, the estrogen level falls and the progesterone level rises. If the egg is not fertilized and implanted, the progesterone level drops abruptly, causing the lining of the uterus to break off and menstruation to begin.

The mood swings caused by these monthly hormonal changes can be unpredictable. Irritability and discomfort can be a problem whenever there is an imbalance of hormones, such as premenstrually, after childbirth, while using birth control pills, and just before menopause, when the ovaries no longer produce eggs and the cycles are less regular. Many

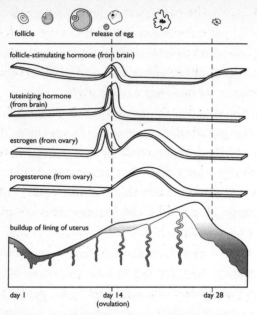

follicle   release of egg

follicle-stimulating hormone (from brain)

luteinizing hormone
(from brain)

estrogen (from ovary)

progesterone (from ovary)

buildup of lining of uterus

day 1   day 14   day 28
                       (ovulation)

Hormone levels and the menstrual cycle

women inherit a particular sensitivity to these hormone changes, and can even develop major depression. Upsetting and stressful events can aggravate this sensitivity.

Premenstrual Dysphoric Disorder

When Katie was feeling all right, she was fun to be around. About seven days before the onset of her period each month, though, her character changed completely. She became abrasive and cutting, and belittled her husband's sexual performance and earning capacity. Finally, he said that he couldn't bear her attacks anymore, and threatened to leave her if she didn't get help. Katie was stunned by his reaction because she hadn't realized how hurtful her attacks were; at the time she always felt that her criticisms were completely legitimate.

When she was in the early part of her cycle, she felt calm and content and pleased with her life. Only in the week before her period did she start to feel edgy, bloated and unattractive. At that stage, any slight joke her husband made would infuriate her, and she would be ready to do battle.

With her husband's ultimatum, Katie decided that she had to do something about her moods. She went to her family doctor, who asked her to chart her moods for three months and coordinate them with her menstrual cycle. She soon noticed that she became irritable within five days of the onset of her period, almost like clockwork. This meant that, by watching the calendar, she could allow for the bad times. She tried not to overextend herself at that time of month. She would book any dinner parties and community work for her calm three weeks. She made sure she got adequate rest and extra help around the house, from her husband and children, during the bad week. She also made a point of looking after herself. She took the dog for a walk each evening. She cut down on coffee and alcohol, as they made her more irritable. She loved to sit in a hot bath in the evenings to unwind. She also treated herself and her husband to a restaurant meal where they could relax without the kids. She was careful to drink lots of water, decrease her salt intake, and eat fresh fruits and vegetables. She took a vitamin B6 pill each morning because she had read that this would help. She also tried positive self-talk such as 'This is just a temporary situation', and 'I know I can get through this'. Her explosions lessened and Katie felt much less stressed out. As for her husband, he tried to be more caring and loving during the rough times. Katie asked him to try this all month long!

Katie had a classic case of premenstrual dysphoric disorder, a variant of depression caused by premenstrual alteration in the balance of estrogen and progesterone. (Premenstrual dysphoric disorder is also known as premenstrual syndrome, or PMS.) This illness is stable and recurrent, marked by anxiety, irritability, mood changes and physical discomfort. The symptoms start five to seven days before the onset of the period and ease up when the period starts. You feel fine until something unexpected happens, and then you explode like a firecracker. The disorder can be managed supportively, by eliminating coffee and alcohol from your diet, relaxing and exercising more, and adding vitamin B6 at a dose of 50 to 500 mg daily, for seven to ten days before your period starts. A diuretic such as bendrofluozide, a medication that increases urine output if there is bloating and water retention, sometimes helps. Your doctor can prescribe it.

Discuss what's happening with your doctor. You might look at areas of stress in your life that can be minimized. You may need to do less during this time of month, or spend more time on activities you enjoy. You may feel it's more 'womanly' to be all-giving and to neglect your own needs, but in the long run this tactic can backfire. Ask for help from your partner or other family members.

About 5 per cent of women with this disorder benefit from psychotherapy and antidepressants. Another 38 per cent also suffer from seasonal affective disorder. A severe form of premenstrual dysphoric disorder can develop if you were sexually abused as a child.

Birth Control Pills

Birth control pills imitate the menstrual cycle by supplying estrogen and progesterone for the first twenty-one days of the cycle. No egg is produced so you can't get pregnant. If

---

Drugs and pregnancy

The safety of various drugs during pregnancy is not well documented. Pregnant women are not included in drug trials, for ethical and legal reasons. Since 1962, when the tranquilizer thalidomide was prescribed for pregnant women in Europe and Canada and babies were born with phocomelia (poorly developed arms and legs), doctors have been reluctant to prescribe any medication during pregnancy, and pregnant women have been wary of taking drugs.

While such caution is understandable, it's also worth remembering that only 30 per cent of drugs are thought to cause birth defects. SSRIs have not been shown to cause such defects, and not treating the mother can be damaging to her health.

Your GP can supply information about the safety of drugs during pregnancy and these are also listed in the British National Formulary (available for purchase in book form or on line at www.bnf.org.uk). For more information, see Further Resources, at the end of this book.

---

you have experienced depression or premenstrual dysphoric disorder, you may be susceptible to the mood alterations these pills produce. Drug manufacturers have tried to alter the dosages of the hormones so that the mood upset is less but ovulation is still prevented.

Pregnancy

Nearly 50 per cent of women experience some level of depression during pregnancy. Unfortunately, only half of this group seek or receive treatment.

ANTIDEPRESSANT DRUGS AND PREGNANCY

Whether you develop depression during pregnancy, or you have pre-existing depression or bipolar disorder, medication can be risky for your unborn child. Lithium, valproic acid and carbamazepine are all known to affect the neurological and physical development of the fetus. Fluoxetine has not been shown to cause problems. Nonetheless, it is probably best not to use any medication in the first three months. If you are taking any of these medications, consult your doctor as soon as your pregnancy is confirmed. Even better, if you are planning to become pregnant, consult your doctor first so that the two of you can plan accordingly, to balance the benefits of protecting your baby against the risks to your mental health. The good news is that, if you have suffered from a depressive disorder prior to getting pregnant, you may notice an improvement in your mood, and less need for medication.

Post-Partum Depressive Illnesses

'Post partum' refers to the first year after childbirth. The levels of the sex hormones fall abruptly at delivery. If you are sensitive to the effects of estrogen and progesterone changes, you may develop mood disorders at this point.

POST-PARTUM 'BLUES'

After your baby is born, you may experience 'blues', feeling weepy and sad for the first two to three days. Support and reassurance are usually enough to get you past this time. Caring and love from your partner and family help as well. Don't expect to be a super-mum! Get plenty of sleep when you can, and don't pretend to feel great if you don't.

POST-PARTUM DEPRESSION

Sarah had been looking forward to the birth of her first son. She had married late and become pregnant soon after her

---

Risk factors for post-partum depression
- fertility problems
- psychiatric illness
- family history of post-partum depression
- being a single parent
- financial difficulties
- being an adolescent mother
- being a mother over thirty-five
- worries about the health of your newborn
- difficult labour
- premature baby
- social isolation
- marital problems

---

honeymoon. When she gave birth to a premature daughter, she was disturbed to realize that motherhood was not what she had fantasized. She couldn't decide on a name for her daughter, and didn't feel any great love for the infant. In fact, she felt flat and uninterested in the people around her, including her husband. She fed the baby with a bottle, as she couldn't tolerate the infant sucking her breast. She was ashamed of herself, and hated the baby, and felt unnatural as a mother.

Sarah didn't want anyone, even her husband, to know what an awful person she was, so she hid her tears and moodiness and tried to pretend she could manage, although she was having terrifying dreams about harming the baby. She finally confided to her best friend, who was a doctor, how miserable she was feeling. Her friend told her that she was probably suffering from post-partum depression, and arranged for Sarah and her husband to see a psychiatrist. Sarah's husband spent more time at home until Sarah started to feel better, and he and her mother agreed to give the baby her bottle during the night so Sarah could get some uninterrupted sleep. She began taking an antidepressant, and had psychotherapy sessions to talk about the pressures she was feeling. Sarah was reassured that she and her husband could get a babysitter and go out for the evening; she had been worried that she had to be on call twenty-four hours a day, because the baby was premature and never slept more than two hours at a time. At last report, Sarah had begun to enjoy playing with her new little girl, and they looked like a happy pair.

If you are among the 10 per cent of new mothers who develop a clinical depression after a week or two or, less often, over the first three or four months, you may require treatment. The depression can interfere with your attachment to your new baby. Sometimes you and your doctor can predict this sensitivity if you have had problems with premenstrual tension or birth control pills, or if you or a close relative previously had a bout of post-partum depression. A loving relationship with a partner helps buffer the effects. Let up on your expectations of yourself, ask for help if you need it, and get adequate sleep.

Antidepressants from the SSRI group can be safely prescribed for you while you are breastfeeding, as there is very little risk to the baby. If you are on lithium it's important to stop breastfeeding, because babies are very sensitive to its effects. If your depression is caused by changes in hormone levels, you will probably respond well to antidepressants. But other changes in your life at this time, such as leaving work, tension in the family, financial worries, sleepless nights, and exhaustion, may aggravate the depression.

POST-PARTUM PSYCHOSIS

This is the most serious type of post-partum depression. It occurs following about one birth in 500, but a woman who has had a bout of post-partum psychosis after one birth has one chance in three of developing another after the next birth.

Psychosis is defined as a loss of contact with reality, often accompanied by frightening delusions and hallucinations. The mother may never have experienced a mental illness before. Some three to fourteen days after the birth, she becomes agitated and confused, with *depersonalization* (feeling detached and outside her body) and insomnia quickly leading to *delirium* (a state of altered consciousness in which she is confused, and disoriented about her identity and the place and time). The striking feature of this illness is its variability; periods of calmness and lucidity can be quickly followed by dangerous, unpredictable actions. She is likely to have auditory hallucinations in which she 'hears' terrifying things.

Post-partum psychosis is a grave *psychiatric emergency*. The mother almost always requires treatment in a safe setting where she can be monitored constantly. When women in this condition are not treated, there is a 4 per cent chance that they will kill their newborns.

Perimenopause and Depression

Don't be surprised if you notice changes in your mood as you approach menopause. During the five to seven years before your periods stop for good, your hormone levels start to change, your periods become less regular, and you may start to have symptoms such as hot flushes, irritability and difficulty sleeping through the night.

According to folklore, serious depression starts at this age, supposedly because women feel 'useless' when they lose their fertility. Statistics don't support this notion; in fact, many women are relieved to leave their child-bearing years behind, and move on to more freedom. All the same, mood changes should be expected. Physical changes such as vaginal dryness and lack of sexual interest may cause irritability. Changes in hormones, and in your sensitivity to them, may cause increased worry and fatigue, and less ability to cope. They won't actually cause depression, but they may change the severity of an existing disorder. For example, bipolar disease may not be recognized until the perimenopause. In women who have bipolar illness, the rapid cycling form often begins around this time.

If you have experienced a mood disorder with a pregnancy or on birth control pills, you are more likely to develop a mood disorder when your sex hormone levels change at menopause, and you may require antidepressant treatment. Hormone replacement therapy (HRT) with estrogen and progesterone supplements can also help. HRT doesn't treat the depression, but it does enhance the effects of any antidepressant medication you may be taking. There has recently been some concern about the safety of HRT. The Committee on the Safety of Medicines advises that use of HRT for more than five years slightly increases the risk of breast cancer. This is something you may wish to discuss with your doctor.

Other changes in your life often happen during the same years as menopause. Children are getting married, going to university, or otherwise leaving home. Elderly parents may need more time and care. Your relationship with your partner may be altering as you both look toward retirement and what you want to accomplish in your remaining time. As women age, of course, they are more likely to lose their partners. About 20 per cent of women who are widowed after age sixty develop depression. If the loss is unexpected or results in decreased financial and emotional security, depression is even more likely to develop.

Having Children, Losing Children

Although the following events and situations usually affect both partners, women generally bear the major impact. However, a loving, supportive relationship can help them weather the changes, so that neither partner develops a depression.

Mothering

Mothering requires a high emotional involvement, but restricts your freedom to plan your life as you please. If you are already vulnerable because of poor education, low self-esteem or a troubled marital state, you are more prone to develop depression. Serious social problems such as job loss, poor housing, overcrowding, threats of eviction, and physical danger can escalate the stress you feel. Twenty-five to 40 per cent of mothers studied in a working-class district of London, with children under six years old, were found to be depressed.

Single parents have added stresses. Finances are often limited. Ongoing disputes with ex-spouses can be exhausting. Juggling the demands of children and a job, as well as running a household by yourself, calls for creative strategies. According to a recent study carried out by

McMaster University in Ontario, Canada, low-income adolescent mothers living on their own are the most vulnerable group, with a 45 per cent incidence of depression.

What will help you survive these years? Practical and emotional support from family and friends, and an intimate relationship with your partner, if you have one, protect you from developing depression. Employment outside the home is also protective, because you develop an increased sense of competence, stimulation and social status. (The money comes in handy, too!) Other practical ways to combat depression might include participating in playgroups with mothers and toddlers at a parent resource centre, or sharing babysitting with other parents so you can both get a night out without children. Local gyms often provide babysitting services while you enjoy working out and talking to other mothers. Informal arrangements with relatives can also give you time for yourself.

Rita was pregnant again, though her first two children were still preschoolers. Her husband, Robert, ran his own plumbing business; he was in and out of the house at all hours and couldn't be depended on to babysit the kids. Rita found herself becoming more and more irritable and tired. Her own family was in Spain for most of the year. Her mother-in-law lived two blocks away and was retired, but they had never been close, because Robert had left his first wife to be with Rita, and her mother-in-law had never approved. Finally, one afternoon when her mother-in-law dropped by for coffee and found the house in a shambles, Rita burst into tears. To her surprise, her mother-in-law said she remembered how tough it had been when she was a young mother. She gave Rita a hug and told her to go and lie down while she cleaned up. After that, Rita and Robert's mother could talk about how they really felt. It turned out that Robert's mother loved helping out with the children, but had felt she would be interfering if she offered to do so. With help from her new-found ally, and antidepressants and therapy from her doctor, Rita found her load much lighter.

In many cultures, there are rituals surrounding childbirth that support the new mother. Women in our own culture have reinstated some of these rituals with childbirth classes, home births, midwives, and husbands taking a more active role. But the most important step is recognizing that depression is not unusual, and that it's all right to ask for help.

Elective Abortion

On the one hand, having an unwanted child causes anguish for everyone. On the other hand, feelings can change over time; even if the decision to have an elective abortion is clear at the time, it may be regretted later. Choosing abortion is probably one of the most difficult decisions a woman ever makes. Pressures from family members, moral teachings, economic needs, and the state of the relationship with the child's father may all influence the decision.

An abortion is much safer in the first three months of pregnancy than later. Because of this time constraint, you may feel you can't make a well-thought-out decision. Teenage girls, who usually have less financial independence, have even fewer options than older women, and may be pressured into making decisions they regret later. Terminating a pregnancy creates a serious and painful loss, but raising an unwanted child can be devastating for both you and your child. It's very important to talk to someone who can be objective if you are doubtful about your decision; speak with your family doctor, or arrange to see a counsellor through a birth control clinic or the outpatient department of a general hospital. A middle ground is to carry the child to term and then give the baby up for adoption. Recently it has become more common for the birth mother and the adoptive mother to stay in contact after the adoption, which often softens the pain of separation for the birth mother.

You can talk with a woman who has been through a similar experience, and she can tell you how she dealt with the pros and cons of these choices. It may also be helpful to talk to friends who have managed to raise a child in difficult circumstances, and find out how they coped. If you have strong religious scruples, it may be helpful to discuss the situation with someone who shares your belief system. Support from your family or your partner can help influence your decision as well.

It is fortunately much less difficult to arrange an abortion now than it was in the past. But that doesn't make it an easy decision. Ten per cent of women develop depression within two years after having an elective abortion.

Infertility

Having difficulty conceiving can be emotionally draining for you and your partner. Generally speaking, if you have tried for a year without any luck, you should start looking for the reasons. About 50 per cent of women who have difficulty do conceive eventually. Infertility has doubled since the 1970s, and about 10 to 15 per cent of couples now cannot conceive without help. Factors in the man, in the woman, or in both can be responsible. The investigations into the reasons are lengthy and difficult and can interfere with your enjoyment of sex. You may lose heart about ever having a child, and may find yourself avoiding family and friends with children as a result.

Treatments for infertility are covered by the NHS to a limited degree as assessed on an individual basis. If your hormone levels are not high enough, you may be given steroids that can affect your mood. The next stages of treatment, through artificial insemination or fertilizing the eggs outside the uterus, can be very frustrating as well, demanding time as well as money, and the chances of success are only about 20 per cent at best.

If these techniques also fail, you may decide to adopt. You then have to be screened by an adoption counsellor, to try to make certain you would be good parents. Lately, fewer newborns have been available – single mothers have been keeping their babies, as the social stigma has lessened – so if you are seeking an infant you may have to go to orphanages in Russia, Romania, China or South America. The costs of travelling and legal and bureaucratic expenses can be very high. All in all, the financial and emotional complexities for you and your partner can cause great distress, especially if one of you would just as soon remain childless.

Even if you do adopt, you may still grieve for a natural child of your own. If you badly wanted children, not having your own child can be a major loss. Moreover, relatives and friends may never accept the adopted child as part of the family. Any of these factors can lead to depression in you or your partner.

Maggie and James had married in their late thirties. They very much wanted a child. Unfortunately, Maggie had severe endometriosis that caused excruciating pain during her periods. She had had an operation and had been placed on hormones to control the pain. She was unable to conceive. She had a history of depression, and her inability to conceive and the effects of the hormone made her depression worse. James started to worry that she would never pull out of it.

They talked to the gynaecologist, who finally stopped the medication; Maggie used painkillers during her periods instead. She gradually started to feel less depressed, but was still devastated at being unable to have a baby. She and James found out all they could about adopting overseas, because they were unable to arrange a local adoption. After many frustrating delays, heavy costs and bureaucratic tangles, James and Maggie adopted a little girl from China.

The next year was also stressful, as the child adapted slowly and they often worried about her physical and mental health. Fortunately, everything turned out well. After a year of devoted parenting, James and Maggie had a delightful, happy little girl who was curious and affectionate. But for many couples, this expensive solution is not an option.

Other Factors of Women's Psychology

Rumination

When women have problems, they tend to ruminate on them, rather than distracting themselves; that is, they think and talk about their problems over and over, to try to come to grips with them. This can work against them taking action, and can cause a downward spiral in their thinking. They may end up feeling hopeless and helpless.

If you find yourself chewing over a problem and not

resolving anything, see if you can step back from it. Consider your options realistically and try to keep the matter in perspective. It may help to write down the positive and negative aspects of various solutions. Fussing never fixed anything!

Body Image

Another area that can increase women's predisposition to depression is body image. Depression seems to develop in girls who are dissatisfied or embarrassed about their appearance. One study showed that girls who experience an obsession with thinness in year 7 are more likely to go on to develop depression as adults. Concerns about body size and attractiveness preoccupy many women.

Fortunately, there's a backlash today against these obsessions and preoccupations. There are some very sensible magazine articles and books about body image and self-respect. Talk to friends, and check your local bookshop or library.

Sexual Abuse

Six to 16 per cent of girls experience unwanted sexual contact before the age of eighteen. Although sexual abuse happens to both boys and girls, it is six times more frequent in girls; boys tend to experience more physical abuse. Early trauma like sexual abuse can cause actual changes in neurological development, 'hot-wiring' the developing brain so that, in later life, the victim over-responds to stimuli; the result can be a permanent state of high arousal and unstable mood.

You are more likely to develop depression as an adult if you have been sexually molested as a child. If you feel that some of your worries are due to molestation, it's important to get counselling; there's no need to carry this burden for the rest of your life. Talk to your doctor or religious advisor.

Spousal Abuse

Women who are being physically abused by their partners often visit their family doctors complaining of depression. Only when asked directly will they confide that they are being abused. Help is available if you are in an abusive relationship, even if you have children and are financially dependent on your partner. Most communities operate shelters for abused women and their children that provide safety, counselling and legal advice. Look in the phone book or ask your family doctor, your religious advisor, or the police for the location of a suitable shelter. The police can also provide protection, in various ways, if you are being threatened or assaulted by a former partner.

10
Depression in the Elderly

Bob is a retired secondary school mathematics teacher. He and his wife, Betty, who live in East Sussex, have three grown children, but they don't see them often. Two of their children are working overseas and the third lives in Scotland, and Bob and Betty can't afford to travel as much as they'd like to.

Shortly after he left his job, Bob developed nerve deafness in both ears that so far can't be improved with a hearing aid. He tried to learn to lipread, but found it difficult because he is nearsighted and doesn't like using glasses. Betty has osteoarthritis that restricts her mobility, so Bob does most of the housework, including the cooking.

Over a period of two months, Bob started to have difficulty sleeping. He woke up every two or three hours during the night, and by four in the morning he was wide awake and couldn't get back to sleep. He had pains in his stomach after he ate that made him think he had cancer, but he didn't want to upset Betty, so kept it to himself. He had difficulty remembering where he had put things, and what to buy at the grocery shop when he got there. The cooking and housework seemed like more and more of a burden. He didn't know how he and Betty would manage in their house as they got older, yet he hated the thought of moving into sheltered housing. He worried about this constantly when he awoke at night.

Bob finally spoke to his doctor about his fear of having cancer. The doctor did a series of tests, including blood tests and an electrocardiogram as well as an ultrasound of Bob's abdomen. He reassured him that there was no sign of cancer. Fortunately, his doctor has elderly parents and is sympathetic to the needs of the elderly; he arranged to have a local community agency provide in-home help three hours a day, as well as a noontime meal, so Bob and Betty could have a hot lunch. The doctor also suggested that Bob try antidepressants to improve his low mood.

With fewer household chores looming over him, Bob decided he could spend some time on his own interests. He had always been intrigued by stories he had heard of some of his ancestors, Huguenots who emigrated from France and settled in Sussex. He decided to take a course in local history and delve into the past. He joined a local historical society, and he and Betty made several new friendships.

Currently, the average lifespan at birth is seventy-six years. At the beginning of the twentieth century it was only forty-six. In fact, you now have a twenty times greater chance of living to one hundred than if you had been born in 1900. Infectious diseases are easily treated in most cases, and nutrition in Western countries has greatly improved. Blood pressure medications are helping to control the frequency of heart attacks and strokes. New diagnostic and surgical

How old is elderly?
For research and statistical purposes, an elderly person is arbitrarily defined as someone sixty-five or older. In medical treatment, though, signs of the individual's physical and psychological aging are more meaningful.

techniques let us deal with many problems before they are life-threatening.

Sometimes, when we're young, we see the elderly as unhappy and lonely, with little reason to live. Fear of our own old age probably clouds our view, leading us to stereotype the old as depressed. In fact, depression occurs less in the elderly than in the young. It may be that, as we age, we are more able to cope with changes because of our life experiences.

Statistics about the depressed elderly are not readily available, because researchers have trouble getting a 'clean' sample to study; illnesses, loneliness, physical restrictions, and the deaths of family and friends are common by the time we reach old age, and all of these complicate the picture. Yet major depression occurs in only 5 to 10 per cent of the healthy elderly. According to a large American study, even people who had recurrent depression as younger adults are less likely to have an episode in old age. When depression occurs for the first time in old age, it's important to look for a physical cause.

Symptoms of depression in the elderly can be different from those in younger people. When you are elderly, you don't often speak of feeling sad or depressed. Depression is less likely to show up as guilt and self-blame. Instead, you may be irritable; you may worry too much, and complain of numerous physical discomforts, such as headaches, muscle pains, stomach troubles, constipation, weight loss and sleeping troubles. You may feel confused, slow in your thinking, forgetful, and not very interested in your family and friends. You may even express indirect suicidal thoughts, such as 'Why am I still here?' or 'I'd be better off dead.'

As we age, we face physical and psychological changes. We may lose the intimate partner who has been our best supporter. We may see less of neighbours and friends because we don't get out as much. We probably no longer work, so we miss out on sharing news and gossip with younger colleagues. Children and grandchildren tell us less, to 'protect' us. We may have less power and status. Loss of hearing, sight and mobility make us more dependent on family members. Our sexual experiences change in scope and frequency. Memory loss worries us.

Living alone is isolating, but living in a residential facility can be demeaning and restrictive. Fear of further disabilities and restrictions leaves us frightened about the future. Having to look after a partner who is suffering from disabilities or dementia may leave us exhausted and depleted, but placing this loved partner outside the home causes us great anguish.

People who had difficulty coping with change and with other people's idiosyncrasies in the past are likely to have even greater difficulties as they age. Those who are content and comfortable physically are more likely to avoid despair in later years.

Being elderly doesn't always mean being inactive. Increased leisure gives you time to investigate interests you always wished you could explore. Late-life learning in areas you've enjoyed, such as music or art, is available, usually at lower rates, from community colleges and universities. Perhaps the skills you used during your paid work can be turned to volunteer work; for example, one retired businessman developed management plans for public agencies that couldn't afford a paid consultant. Staying involved by volunteering at the local daycare, hospital or seniors' club can also be enjoyable. You may find it meaningful to write an informal autobiography, a wonderful legacy for your grandchildren. Keeping fit by walking or working out at a gym will increase your stamina, and may also keep your spirits up. The Internet and e-mail are fantastic for staying in touch. (Your grandchildren can teach you to use the Internet, if necessary.) Many people find support from spiritual and religious communities, as well.

Physical Illnesses and Surgery

Depressive symptoms are part of many physical illnesses that are associated with aging. In yet other physical illnesses, the depression results from the limitations and discomfort the illness causes. If you and your family are told to expect some depression with these illnesses, you may feel less alarmed when it happens.

Heart Attacks and Bypass Surgery

Arteries are the vessels that carry blood with oxygen from the heart and lungs to all parts of the body, including the brain. Our cells require a steady supply of this oxygen in order to do their work. A lack of blood flow for more than four minutes can kill the cells of the body and brain. With aging, however, the walls of the arteries become narrowed with cholesterol deposits, just as sediment can build up inside plumbing pipes. When the buildup is large enough, or if a plug or blood clot blocks the narrowed artery, the artery is no longer able to supply blood to the cells.

A heart attack occurs when the arteries that supply blood to the muscle of the heart itself are blocked, and an area of cells in the heart muscle dies because of the lack of oxygen. Although a major heart attack may be immediately fatal, many people survive lesser heart attacks, and their hearts continue to function despite the damaged area of muscle. But when someone has had a heart attack, the risk of developing depression can be as high as 15 to 20 per cent. The shock of such a close brush with death can be terrifying. You are forced to take stock of the stresses in your life, and decide what is important to you. It's upsetting to realize that, if you don't make substantial changes in your lifestyle, you may die very soon. Joining a rehabilitation and exercise programme on your doctor's advice and talking to someone about your fears can be helpful.

Sometimes, after a heart attack or even before, your doctor may recommend bypass surgery. In this operation, unblocked veins from the leg are transplanted to the heart to replace damaged arteries. This procedure brings a better supply of blood and oxygen to the heart muscle, which helps the heart function better. Despite this improvement, almost 40 per cent of bypass patients develop clinical depression after the procedure. In the first year after surgery, this depressed group has three to four times more risk of dying than the people who do not develop depression after the surgery. We don't know why there is such a high rate of depression, but treatment with adequate doses of antidepressants can help.

Post-Stroke Syndrome

Just as a heart attack is a loss of blood and oxygen to heart cells, a stroke is a loss of blood and oxygen to brain cells. Frequently, a stroke cuts off the blood supply to the left frontal lobe of the brain (the centre for mood regulation), which can result in depression. This is because the damage to the cells of the frontal lobe impairs the smooth operation of functions needed to regulate moods. If you develop depression early in the period after a stroke, antidepressants can alleviate these effects and help speed your recovery. Even if the depression is not directly caused by the stroke, it may develop later if you have decreased ability to move, or difficulty making yourself understood.

Parkinson's Disease

Parkinson's disease is a hereditary illness that usually begins in people sixty or older. It is characterized by tremors, a shuffling gait and a flat facial expression. The hands perform rapid 'pill rolling' movements at rest. Damage to the part of the brain that makes muscle movements smooth and coordinated causes this illness, but the illness doesn't only involve movement. In 50 per cent of cases there is also depression, which is thought to be directly due to the underlying brain damage. Often, though, the person with Parkinson's – and perhaps the family, too – misunderstands the irritability. They don't realize that it's due to depression, but see it as a personality problem. Treating the depression can help.

Vitamin Deficiencies

As it ages, the human body begins to have difficulty absorbing certain nutrients. Decreased supplies of these nutrients going to the brain can cause depression. A doctor who suspects vitamin B12 deficiency or folic acid deficiency generally checks for anaemia, but in 33 per cent of cases the depression begins before the anaemia, so the deficiency may not be recognized for a while. Other blood tests can pick up these specific deficiencies so that supplementary treatment can begin earlier.

Cancer

Depressive symptoms can be an early sign of cancer, before the cancer itself can be detected. A depression that doesn't respond to treatment may be a signal that a brain tumour or pancreatic cancer is present.

Farouk was sixty-seven, and he had worked in the office of an industrial firm until he retired. He was in his second marriage, and he and his wife had a son who was twelve. The couple met jointly with a therapist to talk about the troubled state of their marriage, and Farouk's increasing unhappiness and lethargy. Talking about these problems didn't change Farouk's feelings, so the therapist started him on antidepressants, and began to explore his earlier life. The depression continued, and Farouk developed abdominal pain and began to lose weight. Both his therapist and his doctor felt that the weight loss was probably due to the depression. When Farouk's stomach pains became intolerable, an ultrasound was done, and advanced pancreatic cancer was diagnosed.

Cancer patients often develop depression during the course

of treatment. The loss of function, the uncertainty about the outcome, the fear of painful treatments, and the possibility of dying all contribute to this. Some anti-cancer drugs are also known to cause depression. Doctors and staff of cancer treatment centres are aware of these difficulties, and can offer supportive counselling for the patient and the family, as well as antidepressant therapy. Sometimes the anti-cancer drugs can be changed to ease the symptoms.

If you have cancer, though, sadness and grieving are to be expected. Talking about your fears and having a realistic knowledge of the type of cancer and the prognosis may help. Unfortunately, friends and family sometimes shy away from such discussions because of their own discomfort. This can leave you feeling more lonely and isolated than ever. If you can take a matter-of-fact approach, they may be more able to respond. Consider which facts they probably think would upset you, and speak openly about them. Reassure them that you'd feel better talking about the illness, rather than treating it as something too terrible to mention.

You may find another excellent source of support in volunteers who have had the same illness and have learned various ways of dealing with the changes in appearance, energy and mood. Distractions such as exercise and hobbies and just plain having fun can also help.

Cognitive Changes of Aging

Maintaining an active and healthy lifestyle, with exercise and lots of interests, can decrease the effects of aging. Still, memory does decline with age, although recall is usually affected more than recognition. (In other words, the person recognizes the face of a distant acquaintance, but is unable to recall the name.) People tend to exaggerate the amount of their memory loss if they are asked, reporting losses of 50 to 80 per cent when their performance is actually much less impaired. Older people are also slower at problem solving, and require more repetition to learn. Fortunately, they have a wealth of knowledge, experience and wisdom that far outweighs these limitations.

When someone's first episodes of depression occur late in life, the chance of developing dementia is higher than in people who have had recurrent depressive illness throughout their lives. (In dementia there is a permanent, worsening loss of nerve cells, so that intelligence and memory continue to deteriorate.) Ten per cent of people over sixty-five and 50 per cent of people in nursing homes have dementia. Alzheimer's disease is the most common kind of dementia. Someone with Alzheimer's loses mental functions gradually but steadily.

Another kind of dementia, vascular dementia, is caused by repeated mini-strokes. Vascular dementia shows up as a series of abrupt decreases in function, as further mini-strokes cause more damage. Other dementias include those associated with Creutzfeldt-Jakob (mad-cow) disease, Huntingdon's and AIDS.

Dementia and Depression

Dementia and depression are linked in many ways; in fact, distinguishing between the two can sometimes challenge the doctor. Someone with depression may appear confused and slow in thinking, and feel helpless and hopeless, as if 'losing his mind'. Conversely, people with dementia often feel depressed, because they know that their memory and abilities are failing.

Normal memory loss versus dementia

Age-associated memory loss is mild and does not get worse as more time goes by. The following are no cause for alarm:

* trouble remembering names
* difficulty finding the right word
* forgetting where you put things
* poorer concentration than before

The symptoms of dementia are different, and may include the above, but also include:

* decrease in short-term and long-term memory
* decreased abstract or conceptual thinking ability
* decreased judgement
* decreased language and mobility
* agitation, aggression, psychoses, anxiety
* decreased capacity for work and social interactions

Fortunately, when the diagnosis is not clear, treatment for depression can't hurt. In the early stages of dementia, medication may even help. The MAOI group of antidepressants can be used to improve memory and concentration in dementia, while the SSRIs will decrease irritability and aggression. However, these two types of antidepressants cannot be given at the same time.

Vascular Depression

Since the development of new X-ray techniques such as magnetic resonance imaging (MRI), which can give us detailed pictures of the inside of the brain, another type of depression has been identified. Frequently, an MRI in older people with depression shows bright white areas deep in the brain tissue. Researchers think these changes are caused by narrowing of the small arteries that feed blood to these areas of the brain. It may be that the areas affected are connecting fibres that are important in conveying mood messages in the brain. Researchers are trying to find out more about this newly recognized form.

Functional Disabilities

Other physical problems, such as deafness, blindness and immobility from joint diseases, can cause depression because of the limitations they put on someone's life, the obstacles they create and the social isolation that may result. Although there are now many approaches that may help with these problems – from tools such as advanced hearing aids, large-print books and audiobooks, through community resources such as counselling and transit for the disabled – depressed older people are sometimes reluctant to make use of them. It's easy to slip into an attitude of 'I'm too old to bother', or even 'I'm too old for them to bother with'. No matter what your age, talk to the agencies that deal with your problem. You may be surprised by the help they can offer.

Medications

Many medications used to treat high blood pressure, arthritis, stomach problems, cancer, and so on can cause depression as a side effect. The liver contains enzymes that break down foreign substances like medications. When you are older, your liver and kidneys work more slowly, so medications remain in the body longer and side effects are more likely. When there are several foods and medications competing for the same enzyme, the time for the medication to clear the liver is slowed even more, and toxic levels of medication can build up.

Some drugs used for medical illnesses can also cause psychiatric symptoms. Reserpine can cause depression; prednisolone causes mania in some people and depression in others. If caregivers don't recognize that the symptoms are due to the medical treatment, the medication may be continued, causing further difficulties.

One study found that the average elderly person is taking 4.5 prescription and 3.4 off-the-shelf drugs at any one time. Fifty per cent of the elderly in these studies also misused the medications they had been prescribed, causing drug interactions. Elderly women, particularly, often use excessive amounts of minor tranquilizers such as benzodiazepines, repeatedly ordered over the phone, without seeing the doctor again. Benzodiazepines can cause confusion and may lead to car accidents. Combining benzodiazepines and alcohol can be dangerous as well, especially for someone who's driving. Other drugs commonly abused are the painkiller codeine, and meprobamate, another tranquilizer.

People who are taking steroids or non-steroidal anti-inflammatory drugs for arthritis – over 25 per cent of seniors, in one study – often develop depression, anxiety and confusion. Cimetidine, a medication commonly prescribed for stomach problems, can cause confusion and disorientation. It also interacts with other drugs, particularly tricyclics, benzodiazepines, propranolol (used to treat high blood pressure), and theophylline (used to treat asthma), and increases their toxic effects. In fact, many blood pressure medications cause depression as a side effect. Even drugs such as ibuprofen and aspirin, which can be bought without prescription, may be used in excessive amounts and lead to confusion.

How can you protect yourself? Be sure you understand exactly how you're supposed to take each medication, and stick to the instructions. Avoid using nonprescription drugs that you don't really need. Be sure your doctor knows about all the medications you're using, including nonprescription ones. It may also help to buy all your medications from the same chemists, so that the shop has a full record of what you're using. Most of all – when in doubt, ask!

Mania in the Elderly

Mania is the elated or irritable phase of a bipolar disorder. If mania develops for the first time in old age, an underlying physical cause is almost always present; the illness rarely begins in late life.

People experiencing mania need little sleep and don't feel much like eating. They talk rapidly and their thoughts race, often flitting from one topic to another in a disconnected fashion. They may become extremely irritable if someone disagrees with them. They may develop delusions, usually with a grandiose flavour: that someone important is smitten with them, or that they belong to the royal family; these are fixed ideas that have no basis in fact, but they can't be talked out of them. They may also have hallucinations, seeing or hearing things that aren't there. Mania is a psychiatric emergency. Those afflicted require treatment, as they may exhaust themselves if they don't receive medication to calm them down.

Caregiving Responsibilities

About 12 per cent of the overall population is responsible for another person with chronic health problems – for example, aging spouses or parents with Alzheimer's or other debilitating illnesses. Such caregivers are likely to become depressed, especially when faced with limited resources and a lack of support.

When you are not young yourself and you have an adult child with a chronic mental or physical disorder, the relentless nature of the disorder can drive you to despair. You need to find help from friends, spiritual advisors and professionals in the community, and ask other family members to share the responsibility. A support group may give you ideas about setting limits for the ill or disturbed family member, as well as protecting yourself from guilt and exhaustion. Remember – if you don't take care of yourself first, you won't be able to go on caring for someone else.

Some prescription drugs that may cause depression
- *cimetidine* – for gastric reflux, and gastric and duodenal ulcers
- *bromocriptine, levodopa, selegiline* – for Parkinson's disease
- *atenolol, reserpine, doxazosin* – for high blood pressure
- *lorazepam, alprazolam* – for anxiety
- *dexamethasone, prednisolone, hydrocortisone* – for arthritis and collagen diseases
- *codeine, diclofenac, indomethacin* – for pain and inflammation
- *vincristine, methotrexate* – for cancer

Giving Up Independence

In the past, it was common for elderly people to move in with relatives or go to group residences when they could no longer care for themselves. The present trend is to stay in your own home for as long as possible, with community support such as brought-in meals, visiting homemakers and nurses, and outpatient medical care. However, if you are too disabled to manage at home even with this assistance, you may feel residential care or living with a relative is necessary.

Giving up your home can be a very difficult step. The rate of depression among people in nursing homes and seniors' residences is double that of people in their own homes, and the death rate from physical illness is higher as well. As long as you can be cared for in the community and keep your independence, you should do so. If you have to move to a group residence, make sure it's well run, with adequately trained professional staff, and facilities that compensate for your physical restrictions. Location is important too; you should be close to friends and family, and convenient to shopping areas, if possible.

Bereavement

Esther, who is eighty and checks the obituaries daily, reported to her therapist that in the last month three people she had gone to elementary school with had died. She said she couldn't remember so many people dying so often since World War Two.

A single death can leave us sad and bereft for years; repeated multiple losses are devastating. And death is only one of the losses we face. Partners and close family may become chronically disabled and require care. Your stability may be particularly tested if you have been depressed in the past. Research shows that a strong, intimate relationship with the sick person before the illness may protect you from the strain. Staying in contact with friends and neighbours also helps.

If you lose your partner, grieving is a natural response. You may cry, feel agitated and anxious, have trouble sleeping and lose your appetite. The pain and the yearning for the dead person can be overwhelming. You may even feel you are losing your mind. About 20 per cent of widows and widowers develop depression within the first year of their loss. This depression can be medically treated. Sometimes a self-help group with people who have experienced similar losses is helpful. Staying involved in activities and asking for support from friends and family can also help you cope.

Carlos had nursed his wife, Sonia, through the last three years of a severe and progressive Alzheimer's dementia. At first her doctors had thought Sonia was neurotic, but finally Carlos had convinced them that she needed to see a neurologist, and her condition had been diagnosed. Their children were estranged and offered little help – Sonia and their daughter-in-law did not get along – so Carlos continued working during the day and nursing his wife at night. She woke often, and became demanding and unreasonable as the illness progressed. Carlos managed to stay calm, but he felt increasingly alone and angry.

When Sonia died, Carlos felt some relief, but then immediately started to feel guilty. He questioned whether he had done enough to help her. He started to have difficulty sleeping, and began to lose weight. He took early retirement and stayed home and drank most evenings. Finally, a neighbour suggested he attend a bereavement group that another friend had found helpful.

Carlos went to his first session reluctantly; he wasn't sure the others would understand how he was feeling. When an older woman talked frankly about how difficult her husband had become before he died, Carlos realized with great relief that he could describe how he felt without hiding his less charitable feelings. Eventually, he was able to share with the group how much he missed Sonia, and what fun they had had before she became so ill. He even cried the third time he attended, with a mixture of pain and relief, when he talked about how amusing Sonia could be. He slept well for the first time that night. He began planning to visit his son and daughter-in-law and the grandchildren. He was coming to accept the fact that it was fine for him to find joy in his life, even though Sonia was dead.

Treating Depression in the Elderly

Depression in the elderly is treatable. To write off your symptoms as just 'part of getting old' does you a disservice. Your quality of life may be needlessly impaired.

Interpersonal psychotherapy, described in Chapter 5, can be a very helpful intervention if you are mildly depressed. Dealing with losses and bereavement is one of the first tasks of this type of therapy, and loss of functions such as hearing, sight, or mobility can also be explored. Dealing with role transitions such as the change from work to retirement or the onset of a chronic sickness is also part of this therapy. You and your therapist can discuss interpersonal troubles you may have as you become more dependent on your family, or have to move to residential care where irritating rules and restrictions are in place. Your therapist will listen, understand your perspective, and offer support and practical advice in the here and now. This type of therapy is tailor-made to your needs.

If symptoms persist, or if the depression is more severe, antidepressants may be started. Older people tend to tolerate SSRIs well; tricyclics are best avoided because of the effects they can have on conduction in the heart. (See Chapter 6 for more detail on these medications.)

The general principle of drug treatment in the elderly is *start low and go slow*. As explained earlier, the liver and kidneys function more slowly in older people, and therapeutic levels of the drug are reached sooner and last longer. Sometimes the drug is effective at only 10 per cent of the dose recommended for an average adult.

Elderly people tolerate electroconvulsive therapy (ECT) well; see Chapter 6. If the person is suffering from a psychotic depression with delusions and hallucinations, or is suicidal, or does not respond to other treatments, ECT is the treatment of choice. It has the added advantage of being rapid and safe. After a series of six to twelve treatments, the recovery rate is between 50 and 70 per cent. For someone with depression who is not eating or sleeping, ECT is rapid and may be life-preserving. ECT is also indicated for an older person with depression who can't tolerate medication because of high blood pressure, heart problems, toxicity, or poor tolerance of side effects.

11
Suicidal Tendencies and Involuntary Hospitalization

Elaine, who is twenty-three years old, was in a nurse's training programme and lived alone. After a particularly gruelling shift in the A & E department, she returned to her flat to find a message on her answering machine from Peter, whom she had been dating for six months. He said that he was sorry he didn't have the nerve to tell her in person, but he'd decided to move back in with his former girlfriend. Elaine was furious, and felt betrayed. She called her mother and started to cry. Her mother was impatient, saying, 'How do you always manage to pick these losers?' Elaine slammed down the phone; she had never felt so alone and hopeless in her life. She started to drink a bottle of red wine, although she had had no supper and wasn't used to drinking. She began to feel more depressed but less agitated. She got out an almost full bottle of prescription pills, and systematically washed the pills down with the wine.

Fortunately, her mother realized that she had been abrupt, and tried to call back several times. When there was no answer, she drove to Elaine's flat and opened the door with her key. She couldn't wake Elaine, who had passed out on the sofa but was still breathing, so she called for an ambulance and Elaine was rushed to the nearest A & E department. Elaine was roused and encouraged to walk, and was also given an emetic to make her vomit as many of the pills as possible before they were absorbed into her bloodstream. She was then admitted to intensive care for observation, since no one knew how many pills she had taken.

The next day, a psychiatrist interviewed both Elaine and her mother, and realized that there were family difficulties going back a long time. Elaine had felt stress building up and had been sleeping poorly. She had thought of going for help, but was afraid to see a psychiatrist because she thought she would be considered unfit to work as a nurse. Since it wasn't clear that Elaine would have survived if her mother hadn't found her so quickly, Elaine was admitted to the psychiatric unit, to ensure her safety and permit an evaluation of the risk of a further suicide attempt.

Once Elaine was feeling better, bi-weekly therapy sessions were organized in hospital, so that Elaine could develop some trust in her therapist before she was on her own again. She was started on an antidepressant, but was given only enough tablets to last until her next therapy session. Elaine decided to return to work, but arranged to work fewer hours.

All of us feel down in the dumps at times. We can also feel hopeless if nothing seems to work for us. But to

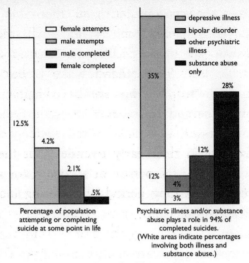

Percentage of population
attempting or completing
suicide at some point in life

Psychiatric illness and/or substance
abuse plays a role in 94% of
completed suicides.
(White areas indicate percentages
involving both illness and
substance abuse.)

Suicide Chart

actually contemplate trying to kill yourself is a very desperate step. People who have reached this state describe their utter despondency and despair, as well as the intolerable suffering they experience. No other solution seems possible to them.

A suicide attempt is a psychiatric emergency. In the UK 3,500 deaths a year are due to suicide. In men under 35 it is the highest cause of death. Women attempt suicide more often than men, but they less often complete the act. Most psychiatric disorders, such as depression, bipolar disorder and substance abuse, are associated with a high risk of suicide. Fifteen per cent of seriously depressed people die by suicide.

Many people who attempt suicide overdose on medication, as Elaine did. Often, alcohol and street drugs that alter the person's judgement are used as well. The incidence of death by suicide has steadily increased since the 1940s.

If you are seriously considering suicide, or if you know anyone who is, get help. Don't try to handle the situation by yourself. At your local A & E department, a doctor can evaluate the risk. Hospitalization may be necessary. Remember that people who are saved after a suicide attempt are often vastly relieved to still be alive. The psychiatric illnesses associated with suicide often begin when people are in their early twenties, but they are not recognized, by either the person or a doctor, for an average of eight years. This long period of suffering increases the risk of suicide – especially since people in this age group have usually left their parents' home, and may not be getting as much emotional support as they had before.

Warning Signs

If you recognize that your friend or relative has a depressive disorder, a bipolar illness, or an alcohol or substance abuse problem, you can help. At some point, 41 per cent of people suffering from depression are suicidal. Most suicides occur

---

Warning signs of suicide
- direct and indirect threats of suicide
- previous attempts at suicide
- family history of suicide
- feelings of depression, hopelessness
- isolation and loneliness
- agitation followed by calm, as if the person has made a decision
- giving away valued possessions
- discussion and preparation of means to commit suicide
- changing a will
- alcohol and substance abuse
- death of a loved one, divorce, job loss, legal trouble

when the person is recovering from depression, six to nine months after leaving hospital. Although people with mental illness have a ten times greater chance of committing suicide over their whole lifespan, most suicides occur in the first three years of the illness. The more likely candidates are younger, have attempted suicide before, have relatives who have attempted suicide, are single or divorced, and show a triad of symptoms: depression, hostility and apathy. Distressing agitation, panic attacks, irritability, and severe anxiety and guilt are usually present just before the act, as well as insomnia and psychotic symptoms. People in mixed bipolar states are quite vulnerable as well.

Emile Durkheim, a French sociologist, coined the term *anomie* to describe the state of a person who is disconnected from the community and at high risk of suicide. People who have values emphasizing connectedness to the community are deterred from committing suicide. Reasons for living, such as responsibility to family, fear of social or moral disapproval, and strong spirituality, also help to deter people from committing suicide.

Ben developed an agitated depression shortly after his father had a stroke that left him speechless. Prior to his marriage, Ben and his father had been close. His father had always been his greatest fan. Since the marriage, however, there had been ongoing friction between Ben's family and his wife's family.

Ben was devastated but felt helpless to make amends with his father now that he was sick. He greatly exaggerated his own responsibility for causing the stroke. Even though people reassured him that his behaviour had not hurt his father, he was unable to get relief. His anxiety became intolerable, and he was hospitalized and placed on tranquilizers. One weekend he had a pass from the hospital and went to visit his parents. After he left their house, he intentionally walked into the path of an oncoming train. He was killed instantly.

Who Commits Suicide?

The tendency to commit suicide is thought to be inherited independently from the tendency to suffer depression. Close relatives of people who have committed suicide are eight times more likely to do so themselves. So anyone who has previously attempted suicide or who has a close relative who has attempted suicide is at high risk. However, it's difficult to decide how much of this risk is due to other factors, such as copying suicidal behaviour and having depressive illness in the family.

Studies have shown that doctors frequently treat people who have attempted suicide inadequately, both before and after the suicide attempt. Sometimes a hospital bed is not available, or a therapist can't be found soon enough. Other times, the stigma around having emotional problems prevents people from getting the help they need.

Suicide attempts are marked by symptoms that occur in depression, but the predisposition to suicide itself seems to have a distinct biochemical and genetic basis. People who are prone to suicide have a lower than usual level of serotonin in the central nervous system. This deficiency is present even when the person is not suicidal.

Perfectionists are another group who are at greater risk of suicide. They set themselves exceedingly high, self-imposed and unrealistic standards, and believe that others expect them to meet impossible goals, and that they will not be accepted if they fall short. This group is prone to both depression and suicide, but they have difficulty accepting treatment because nothing offered ever seems quite good enough. People with personality disorders also have a high risk of suicide.

Cultural beliefs that glorify suicide increase the risk. The Japanese practice of hara-kiri is the classic example. As well, the media publicize the act by talking about celebrities who have committed suicide, such as Jim Morrison. Often there are copycat suicides after someone famous kills himself.

As a preventive measure, professionals and consumer advocacy groups have attempted to advise the media about reporting suicides; they can avoid giving details of how the act was done, and not speculate on the motives of the person who has died. Articles in the media can also help to educate the public about the illnesses that caused this extreme behaviour.

The Emotional Aftermath of Suicide

Someone who commits suicide often leaves relatives and friends bewildered. It's not uncommon for them to feel rage as well as despair. Grieving for a loved one is painful and debilitating at any time; when your feelings are predominantly angry, your grief is even more painful. Close survivors often feel that they should have noticed more, loved more, helped more, done more. The guilt can be consuming. If you didn't notice how depressed the person was, you blame yourself. If you did know but you still couldn't prevent the death, you feel helpless and powerless. In addition, spending time with someone who refuses to take the help offered, and goes on to commit suicide, can leave you feeling not only guilty but also relieved that your exhausting vigilance is no longer required.

How family and friends can help

If someone you know shows signs of potential suicide, here are some steps you can take.

- Take the threats seriously.
- Don't promise confidentiality.
- Get help. Call the person's therapist, or 999, or go to the A & E department of your local hospital.
- Listen and acknowledge the person's feelings. Stay calm and offer reassurance.
- Do not leave the person alone.

This feeling of relief only compounds your guilt. You rework what could have prevented the suicide over and over in your mind, always feeling that you could have done more.

Other people, including professionals, may inadvertently imply that the survivors were somehow negligent and irresponsible. One way and another, the survivors are repeatedly reminded of the desperation their loved one must have felt, to die so tragically and uselessly. The aftermath of a suicide can reverberate for years. Couples break up; family members stop speaking to each other. Children blame themselves for not being more loving or caring to a depressed parent, and parents berate themselves for failing their child in some irrevocable way.

The stigma and blaming connected with mental illness suggest that the act was carried out to punish the survivors for failing the person in some way. This is not the case. The suicidal individual is escaping from intolerable pain. The decision to commit suicide results from a serious distortion of emotional reality, not from a logical choice. Once you recognize that the suicidal act itself is not rational, you can forgive your loved one and yourself, in order to move past this terrible tragedy.

Programmes to Prevent Suicide

Public awareness campaigns in Scandinavia and Hungary have been very successful in lowering the suicide rates. Both places have very high suicide rates, and have mounted public campaigns to educate people to watch for the signs of impending suicide, to know where help is available, and to decrease the stigma and shame. Programmes educating doctors to watch for signs of depression, and to use effective doses of antidepressants, have also helped lower the suicide rates in both places.

At present we can't screen the general population for risk with any accuracy, but we can study high-risk groups to see what interventions work best to reduce the rate. We tend to intervene actively, when someone is seen to be at very high risk, by hospitalizing the individual for his or her own safety. A more long-term and useful approach might be to track people identified as showing suicidal behaviours. With early identification and monitoring, they might be encouraged to seek help sooner. Tracking vulnerable people would be feasible with computer technology; once they had been identified as being at risk, this could be entered on their health files so that any signs of a depressive illness could be treated promptly.

Some of our interventions, such as medication for the treatment of depression, do make a difference in suicide risk. In studies, lithium has been shown to decrease the risk of suicide directly when used to treat bipolar illness. Both the depressed state and the mixed, irritable state of bipolar illness are risky, because of the acute distress the person suffers. In someone who receives lithium, the risk of suicide is 0.37 per cent. Without treatment, the risk is 3.39 per cent.

The increased use of adequate doses of antidepressants to treat major depressive episodes can also decrease the suicide rate. This was shown in the public health campaigns in Scandinavia and Hungary mentioned above. In the United States, the use of antidepressant medication for the treatment of depression increased from 6.5 per cent in 1985 to 68 per cent in 1995. During the same period, the overall suicide rate started to decrease, for the first time since the 1940s. This is a beginning, but we know that depression continues to be both under-reported and under-treated.

Involuntary Hospitalization

Someone who is suicidal and who agrees that he or she needs protection can be admitted by a doctor to a hospital for safety and treatment. The problem arises when someone is judged by a doctor to be suicidal but does not accept this judgement, or does not wish to be helped. In the UK the Mental Health Act defines legal provisions to deal with this situation. The doctor is given temporary powers to overrule the person's wishes, on the understanding that this will ultimately benefit the person.

Anglo-American law does not ordinarily allow preventive detention of someone who may potentially commit a crime but has not yet done so. (Suicide was considered a crime in Canada until 1972 and in the U.S. until 1974.) On one hand, there is a medical and moral duty to protect someone who is seriously planning suicide. On the other hand, people cannot legally be held against their will unless they have given cause. The solution at present is to allow involuntary admission, under specific conditions, within a limited timeframe.

In order to be acting in good faith, a doctor who is hospitalizing someone against his or her will must make the decision based on the following criteria:

- Because of the mental illness, does the person have a decreased ability to make his own decisions?
- Will the person benefit from being hospitalized?
- Is the person a danger to himself or others?

Obviously, all these criteria depend on the good judgement of the doctor.

Involuntary hospitalization is typically instituted if the person is a 'danger to himself or others'. In addition, an appeal procedure is available in the UK for people who believe they have been hospitalized against their will without adequate cause.

Researchers have contacted people, after they recovered, to study their reactions to involuntary hospitalization. More than half of those who initially felt they did not need hospitalization had later changed their minds. They felt more anger about the disrespect and coercion shown by professionals at the time of admission than about the actual hospitalization. They often reported more threats and force being used than were recorded in the doctor's notes. When they were treated with respect and given appropriate explanations, they ended up being much less angry and resentful. Obviously, involuntary hospitalization can save lives – but it must be used carefully, with the appropriate safeguards and reviews, and it will be more effective if the people being treated are given as much consideration as possible.

12
Stigma and Disability

What we don't understand frightens us. It's particularly frightening when something we value as much as our reason and emotions is affected. Our very identity is tied up in trusting the way in which we perceive what happens to us. In the past, explanations of mental illness were often tied to notions of punishment for sins committed, or to bodily possession by demons. Even though we know better now, these myths can still shape our feelings and our fears.

In her book *Illness as Metaphor*, Susan Sontag uses the histories of tuberculosis and cancer as examples of how we perceive illnesses we don't understand. The same principles apply to some of our perceptions of emotional disorders. Sontag says that, when the cause of an illness is a mystery and its effects are alarming, we tend to blame the victim. This person must have committed some offence that brought about the illness – most likely by not following certain civilized rules of behaviour. As soon as a more scientific cause for the illness is found, the illness is seen as being out of the person's control, and the person is no longer blamed.

Most 'psychiatric' illnesses move from the realm of psychiatry (the treatment of medical and emotional problems) to the domain of neurology (the treatment of physical disorders of the brain and central nervous system) when a definite cause is found. Epileptics, with their mysterious seizures, were thought to be possessed by demons until it was found that a scar on the brain surface set off the seizures. Mental retardation was a sign of the gods' disfavour until the many different physical causes were discovered.

As medical science finds biochemical and genetic causes for mental disorders, the stigma attached to them gradually diminishes. But some people still feel – or are made to feel – that they are to blame for their disease. As a result, 50 per cent of people with these disorders do not go for the help they need, and they miss out on effective treatments that would allow them to lead happier, more productive lives.

Scott Simmie and Julia Nunes, two journalists, have published a book called *The Last Taboo*, which describes an episode of mania that Simmie developed after a particularly stressful reporting assignment, and Nunes's attempts to get help for him. Simmie says that one of the most painful aspects of the disease was the lack of acceptance by, and understanding from, his friends and colleagues – *even after* he had recovered. In her book *An Unquiet Mind*, Kay Redfield Jamison, professor of psychiatry at Johns Hopkins University, describes how her colleagues would avoid talking with her about her bipolar I disorder.

When Discrimination Costs Money

Insurance programmes and the workplace are two areas where stigma can be particularly unjust. Insurance plans generally cover psychological treatment to a much lesser extent than treatment for physical illnesses. In the United States, for every dollar spent on serious physical illness, only twenty cents is spent on serious emotional disorders. Private health insurance also discriminates against people with psychiatric problems. Even though many of these are lifelong illnesses, there are ceilings imposed that limit the coverage of drugs and hospitalization available over a lifetime. Once the limit is reached, the drugs are no longer covered and it's difficult to find another insurance company to provide coverage.

In the UK everyone has the right to healthcare, so hospitalization expenses are paid by national healthcare plans. Seniors and people on welfare can receive most prescribed drugs, for a nominal fee. People who are not on welfare but who have no drug plan are responsible for their own drug costs.

Every psychiatrist has stories about patients being discriminated against due to their mental disorder. Joseph was a serious, hard-working man who was being treated for depression with therapy and antidepressants. He had never missed a day of work and had never been hospitalized for depression. When he applied for mortgage insurance on his house, he was turned down because he had truthfully answered 'yes' when asked if he was receiving antidepressants. A physical condition such as high blood pressure can lead to loss of income, yet it's unlikely he would have been denied insurance for taking blood pressure medication.

Telling your employer

Many employers fear increased absenteeism and poorer work performance from employees with psychiatric problems. How can you be honest about your health but minimize the risk of discrimination? The following suggestions are adapted from a 1993 report produced for the US president.

- Choose your timing. After a positive evaluation or after securing a new job is probably the best time to disclose your disorder.
- Focus on the positive aspects of how you cope with the illness.
- Explain the impact of the illness on your job performance, and outline any accommodations that may be necessary.
- Describe your problem as resolved or treated.
- Don't give a psychiatric diagnosis. Use phrases such as 'having difficulties' or 'having a disability and experiencing difficulties'.
- Role-play what you are going to say with a friend or relative.

Discrimination in the workplace has been countered with effective legislation. In 1995 the UK Disability Discrimination Act guaranteed 'accommodation' on the job for people with psychiatric disabilities. For someone who is psychiatrically disabled, accommodation might include such adjustments as flexible working hours, a secluded office with less distraction, and changes in tasks to decrease stress when necessary.

Educating Others

There are many ways to counter discrimination. When you talk to friends and colleagues, be as open as you would be about a disorder like asthma or arthritis; explain the ways you've found to cope, and what has helped and what hasn't. Intervene if prejudicial remarks are made. Write to politicians or the newspapers if you feel you have seen evidence of discrimination. Ask political candidates to talk about what initiatives they are taking to help people with psychiatric disorders. Attitudes do change. For example, homosexuality is now much more widely perceived as normal, after years of political action. If people are made aware that there are effective treatments for psychiatric illnesses, and if the illnesses are demystified, fear and denial gradually decline.

You can also write letters to newspapers and magazines if you feel their reporting has been discriminatory. Praise and promote balanced articles about emotional disorders. Disclosure of their own illnesses by well-known people has helped tremendously. John Cleese, Elizabeth Taylor, Marianne Faithfull and Sinead O'Connor have all been active in describing their struggles with depression and addictions.

Consumer self-help groups and organizations have done tremendous work in decreasing discrimination and empowering people who are psychiatrically ill. MIND, the Depression Alliance, the Mental Health Foundation and many other organizations all provide education, support and advocacy for consumers of mental health services. The goals of consumer groups vary, from increasing the self-esteem of group members to raising public awareness and taking polit-ical action against discriminatory practices.

Disability

In the UK disability is defined by the Disability Discrimination Act as a person who has a mental or physical impairment which causes an adverse effect on their ability to carry out normal day-to-day activities. The adverse effect must be substantial and has lasted, or is likely to last, for more than 12 months.

Average lost years of health from various causes	
	number of DALYs
coronary artery disease	8.9
major depression	6.7
cardiovascular disease	5.0
alcohol use	4.7
traffic accidents	4.3

Since 1990, the World Health Organization has been measuring Disability Adjusted Life Years (DALY) from various causes. The DALY of an illness refers to the average number of healthy years lost from someone's expected lifespan due to premature death, or to the inability to function at home, at work and socially because of a disability. It turns out that the loss from major depressive disorder is second only to that from serious coronary disease. By 2020, major depressive disorder is expected to be the number-one cause.

In the UK legislation protects you from unfairness if you develop a depressive illness while working. Most large companies have sick leave and disability group plans, both short-term and long-term, that cover a portion of your salary if you require time off for a depressive disorder. You will need a statement from a qualified physician, stating the nature of your condition and why you are not able to work. If you have health insurance and the insurance company questions your reasons, you may be asked to see the company's own physician. If there is still disagreement about the claim, you can ask for an independent evaluation of your eligibility.

Private insurance companies make their own rules, and they don't always cover high-risk individuals. (Depressive illnesses are often considered high risk because they may be recurrent and require lengthy treatment.) Unfortunately, no legislation prevents discriminatory practices by insurance companies in terms of whom they will and will not insure.

Sometimes it's hard to remember that you are entitled to the same help for psychiatric disability as you would be for physical disability. Because of discrimination and your own embarrassment, you may not always get the financial assistance and treatment you need. Be persistent and determined in getting your rights. You may want to seek legal advice as well, if necessary.

If you feel you are being discriminated against in the workplace, insist on your rights under the law. If you are having difficulties with your treatment in the NHS or with private insurers, contact a local mental health advocacy group. Considerable progress has been made toward fair treatment for people with psychiatric disorders. Your rights will protect you more, though, if you know what they are.

Conclusion

It can be difficult and discouraging to live with a depressive illness, whether you have the illness yourself, or are helping a loved one cope with the disease. Fortunately, a great deal of exciting scientific research is currently being done to explore the nature of these illnesses, and to discover new treatments. In the next ten years or so, many developments are bound to change the way we view depression, and improve the ways we treat it.

New and intricate technologies – such as the positron emission tomography (PET) scan – are being developed, to allow scientists to see how the brain works in real time. Extraordinary advances in the field of neuroscience will help us understand the changes happening in the brain at a cellular level when someone has a depressive illness.

Recent advances in mapping the genetic code may lead to the identification of specific genetic profiles for these disorders. Some chromosome sites have been discovered in family pedigrees, although they don't explain the defect in all cases.

Remember: depressive illness IS an illness
- It's a common illness; one in five people suffers at least one bout at some time.
- It's debilitating; of all chronic diseases, only heart disease causes more disability and death.
- It's treatable: it responds well to various treatments, yet it's not treated as soon or as often as it should be.
- Treatment that begins early and continues until the person is free of symptoms can decrease the frequency of recurrences and prevent the disease from becoming chronic.

If you're dealing with a depressive illness, don't let attitudes and misconceptions – your own, or other people's – stand in your way. Talk to your doctor and your local mental health association. Talk to your friends and family. Get the help you need.

Developments in pharmacology are paving the way for drugs that are more specific to the illness, and less uncomfortable to take. Three-dimensional computer simulations of drugs can rule out the ones that won't be effective, without unnecessary expense and delay. Some newer technologies, such as transcranial magnetic stimulation (described in Chapter 6), may allow us to treat depressive illness without the invasiveness and risks of drug therapy.

Toward the end of 2001, there were press reports that a nutritional pill containing ingredients used to cure pigs of ear-biting and tail-biting disease also reduced the symptoms of bipolar illness in 55 to 66 per cent of people after six months. Such reports are intriguing, but they call for more study. Before you rush off to the nearest animal feed supplier, remember that the placebo effect may account for half that improvement, and that the natural course of bipolar illness varies greatly.

Finding ways to identify the illness in younger age groups

may help us intervene earlier, before the illness is full-blown. This may even allow prevention; there is evidence that starting treatment early and continuing it for a period of time after symptoms disappear may stop the illness from becoming chronic, as well as forestalling the more disabling symptoms.

While the potential high-tech approaches are dazzling, psychosocial treatments remain essential. Anyone who has been helped in therapy will tell you that, while the medications are useful, the care and insights received in therapy give hope that you can use for your whole life.

In 1992 the Defeat Depression Campaign was launched in the UK – a five-year campaign designed by the Royal College of Psychiatrists and the Royal College of General Practitioners. Its aims were:

1. To educate health professionals, particularly general practitioners about recognizing and treating depression.
2. To educate the general public about depression and the availability of treatment in order to encourage people to seek help earlier.
3. To reduce the stigma associated with depression.

In April 2002 the Department of Health released the consultation document, National Suicide Prevention Strategy for England, laying our strategies to reduce suicide rates in the UK.

Both these reports focused attention on prevention through education, urging that both front-line professionals (doctors, nurses, psychologists, social workers, teachers, clergy, and so on) and the general public be better informed about how depressive illnesses can be diagnosed early and treated effectively. Both reports also emphasized the fact that consumers of mental health services must feel empowered to speak of their needs and experiences, and must press for improved treatment and public awareness.

Since most of us have been touched, directly or indirectly, by these illnesses, there's no reason to feel alone. When people share their experiences through talking and writing, the illnesses become more understandable and less frightening for everyone. There is hope out there. We need to share it.

Table of Drug Names

Generic Name	Some common brand names	Type
amitriptyline	Tryptizol	Tricyclic antidepressants
clomipramine	Anafranil	
dothepin	Prothiaden	
doxepin	Sinequan	
imipramine	Tofranil	
lofepramine	Gamanil	
nortriptyline	Allegron	
citalopram	Cipramil	Selective serotonin reuptake inhibitors (SSRIs)
fluoxetine	Prozac	
paroxetine	Seroxat	
sertraline	Lustral	
isocarboxazid	Marplan	Other antidepressants
mirtazapine	Zispin	
moclobemide	Manerix	

nefazodone	Dutonin	
phenelzine	Nardil	
reboxitine	Edronax	
trazodone	Molipaxin	
venlafaxine	Efexor	
carbamazepine	Tegretol	Mood stabilizers
lamotrigine	Lamictal	
lithium	Camcolit, Liskonum,	
	Priadel	
sodium valporate	Epilim	
valproic acid	Convulex	
chlordiazepoxide	Librium, Tropium	Tranquilizers and sedatives
clonazepam	Rivotril	
diazepam	Valium	
lorazepam	Ativan	
oxazepam	Serenid	
chlorpromazine	Largactil	Antipsychotics
fluphenazine	Moditen, Modecate	
pericyazine	Neulactil	
perphenazine	Fentazin	
propranolol	Inderal	Miscellaneous drugs mentioned in text
trytophan	Optimax	

Glossary

Attention Deficit Hyperactivity Disorder (ADHD): A syndrome beginning in childhood and persisting into adulthood, characterized by distractibility, inattention and hyperactivity.

Bipolar I Disorder: A mood disorder characterized by recurrent bouts of mania and depression.

Bipolar II Disorder: A mood disorder characterized by recurrent bouts of hypomania and depression.

Cyclothymia: A tendency to have mood swings, both high and low, that are less severe than bipolar disorder.

Delirium: An altered state of consciousness with confusion, disorientation and misinterpretation of events. Delirium is usually reversible, and is often due to ingested toxins such as alcohol, or head injury, or a metabolic illness such as diabetes.

Delusion: A false, fixed belief that cannot be changed by reason and is not consistent with the person's cultural background.

Dysthymia: Chronically depressed mood that occurs for most of the day, more days than not, for at least two years.

Emotion: A complex feeling state that has psychological, physical and behavioural aspects.

Endorphins: Chemicals similar to opiates, but produced by the body, to relieve pain.

Enzymes: Catalysts produced by the body that facilitate chemical changes in the brain.

Episode: A single occurrence of a mood disorder.

Feeling: A subjective experience of emotion.

Genetic: Inherited from parents, and passing on physical and behavioural traits.

Hallucination: Sensory perception that occurs without any external cause but seems real to the person experiencing it.

Hypomania: An elevated, expansive, or irritable mood lasting several days, and perhaps years, but not severe enough to cause marked impairment in functioning, to require hospitalization, or to develop into psychosis.

Magnetic Resonance Imaging (MRI): A scan producing an image of the brain by mapping magnetic fields.

Major Depressive Disorder: An illness characterized by repeated bouts of major depressive episodes.

Major Depressive Episode: A clinical depression lasting for six months to two years if untreated.

Maladaptive: Inappropriate or counterproductive; maladaptive behaviour contributes to the risk of developing a psychiatric disorder.

Mania: A psychosis; an abnormal and persistently elevated, expansive, or irritable mood lasting at least one week, with impaired judgement and disconnection from reality.

Manic-Depressive Illness: A synonym for bipolar illness.

Melancholia: A distinct quality of depressed mood

characterized by early morning wakening, agitation or slowed movement, loss of weight, slowed thinking, and excessive or inappropriate guilt.

Mixed Episode: An episode of a mood disorder that includes both manic and depressive symptoms.

Mood: A sustained period of emotion.

Neurotransmitter (NT): A molecule responsible for transmission of a nerve impulse across the synapse between two nerve cells. Serotonin and norepinephrine are neurotransmitters.

Opiate receptors: Cell receptors that pick up either external opiates or internal endorphins to relieve pain and cause euphoria.

Personality: A stable pattern of behaviour that determines how we think about, act in, and see our world.

Pituitary: The central gland at the base of the brain that coordinates the activity of other hormones in the body.

Post-partum: During the first year after childbirth.

Psychodynamics: Explanations of thinking and behaviour based on principles first outlined by Freud and developed by psychoanalysts.

Psychosis: Illness in which the person is out of touch with reality. Often accompanied by delusions and hallucinations.

Rapid Cycling Disorder: A variant of bipolar disorder in which the person has four or more mood swings within one year. The mood swings can be mania, hypomania, or depression severe enough to be considered an episode.

Receptor: A protein configuration on the wall of the receiving cell that a neurotransmitter such as serotonin or norepinephrine can attach to, after the message has crossed the synapse.

Soft Bipolarity: Another name for bipolar II disorder.

Stress: Stimulus causing excessive strain or tension.

Tardive dyskinesia: A permanent movement disorder sometimes occurring after chronic use of anti-psychotic drugs.

Further Resources

Other Websites
Depression Resource Center
www.healingwell.com/depression/
Mayo Clinic Depression and Mood Disorders Page
www.mayohealth.org/home?id=SP3.1.11.5
Suicide Awareness – Voices of Education (SA\VE)
 www.save.org

Books
Baumel, Syd. *Dealing with Depression Naturally*. Lincoln-
  wood, IL: Keats, 2000.
Graham, P. and Hughes, C. *So Young, So Sad, So Listen*.
  London: Gaskell, 1995.
Greenberger, Dennis, and Christine Padesky. *Mind over
  Mood*. New York: Guilford, 1995.
Jamison, Kay Redfield. *Night Falls Fast*. New York: First
  Vintage, 1999.
——. An Unquiet Mind. New York: *First Vintage*, 1996.

Klein, Donald, and Paul Wender. *Understanding Depression.* New York: Oxford University Press, 1993.

Ledoux, Joseph. *The Emotional Brain.* London, UK: Phoenix, 1998.

Lyden, Jacki. *Daughter of the Queen of Sheba.* New York: Penguin, 1997.

McKenzie, Kwame. *Family Doctor Guide to Depression.* London, UK: Dorling Kindersley, 2000.

Millett, Kate. *The Loony-bin Trip.* New York: Touchstone, 1991.

Pitt, B. *Down with Gloom.* London: Gaskell, 1993.

Plath, Sylvia. *The Bell Jar.* London, UK: Faber and Faber, 1963.

Simmie, Scott, and Julia Nunes. *The Last Taboo.* Toronto: McClelland & Stewart, 2001.

Solomon, Andrew. *The Noonday Demon: An Atlas of Depression.* New York: Scribner, 2001.

Styron, William. *Darkness Visible.* New York: First Vintage, 1990.

Wolpert, Lewis. *Malignant Sadness.* London, UK: Faber and Faber, 1999.

Reports
'National Suicide Prevention Strategy' available at
www.doh.gov.uk/mentalhealth

Index